The Joint Commission

AF820754

Treatment Planning in Behavioral Health Care and Human Services

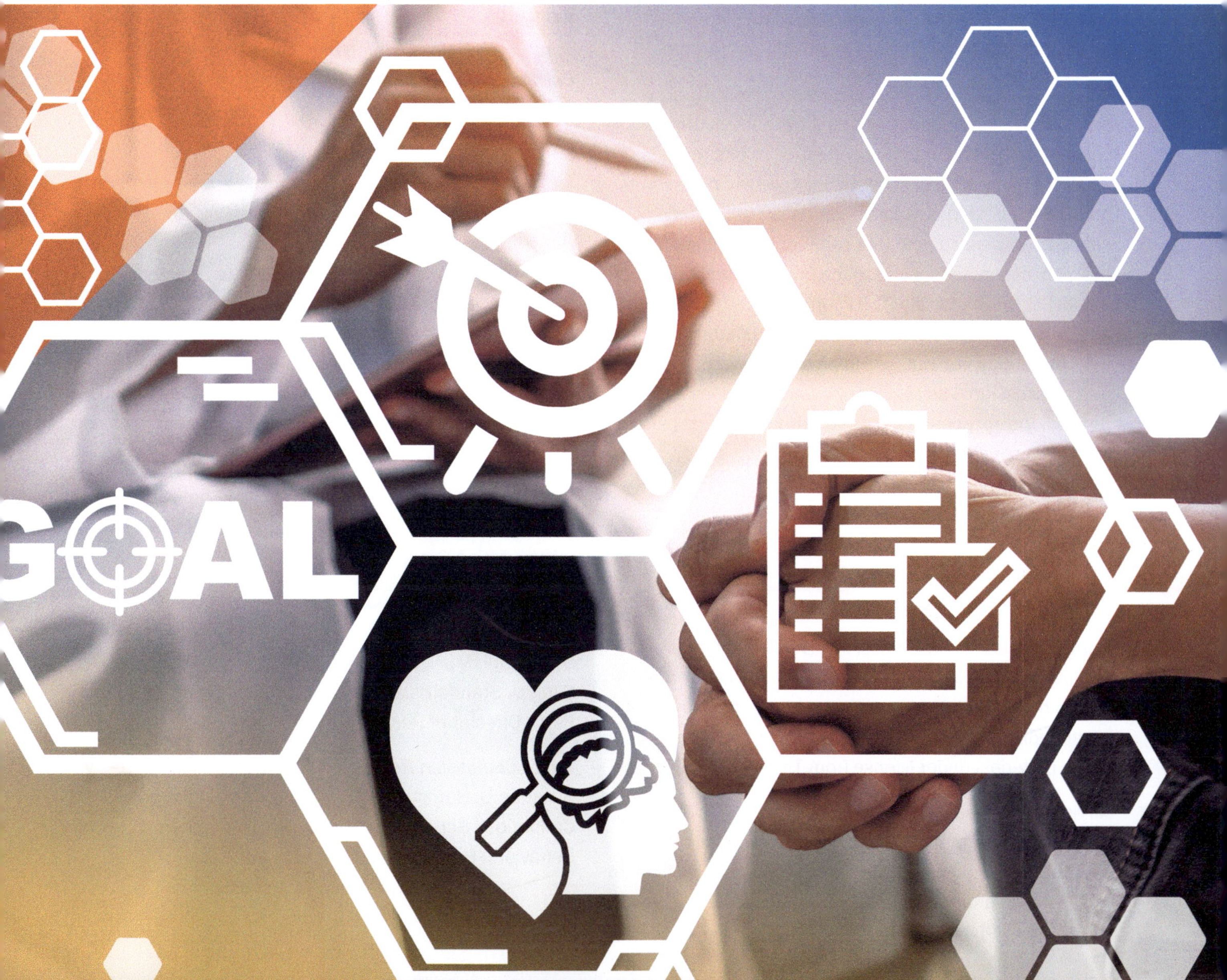

Edited by Jennifer Johnson, MEd, MBA, LPC

Joint Commission Resources Mission

The mission of Joint Commission Resources (JCR) is to continuously improve the safety and quality of health care in the United States and in the international community through the provision of education, publications, consultation, and evaluation services.

Disclaimers

JCR educational programs and publications support, but are separate from, the accreditation activities of The Joint Commission. Attendees at Joint Commission Resources educational programs and purchasers of JCR publications receive no special consideration or treatment in, or confidential information about, the accreditation process. The inclusion of an organization name, product, or service in a JCR publication should not be construed as an endorsement of such organization, product, or service, nor is failure to include an organization name, product, or service to be construed as disapproval.

This publication is designed to provide accurate and authoritative information regarding the subject matter covered. Every attempt has been made to ensure accuracy at the time of publication; however, please note that laws, regulations, and standards are subject to change. Please also note that some of the examples in this publication are specific to the laws and regulations of the locality of the facility. The information and examples in this publication are provided with the understanding that the publisher is not engaged in providing medical, legal, or other professional advice. If any such assistance is desired, the services of a competent professional person should be sought.

Published by Joint Commission Resources
Oak Brook, Illinois 60523 USA
https://www.jcrinc.com

Joint Commission Resources, Inc. (JCR), a not-for-profit affiliate of The Joint Commission, has been designated by The Joint Commission to publish publications and multimedia products. JCR reproduces and distributes these materials under license from The Joint Commission.

ISBN (print): 978-1-63585-226-4
ISBN (e-book): 978-1-63585-227-1

Printed in the USA

For more information about The Joint Commission, please visit **https://www.jointcommission.org**.

Development Team

Associate Director, Books and Digital Subscriptions: Phyllis Crittenden
Editorial Coordinator: Kristine Stejskal
Senior Project Manager: Christopher Zwirek
Associate Director, Production: Johanna Harris
Executive Director, Global Publishing: Catherine Chopp Hinckley, MA, PhD

Reviewers

Joint Commission Division of Accreditation and Certification Operations
Peter Vance, LPCC, CPHQ, Field Director, Behavioral Health Care and Human Services, Surveyor Management and Development

Joint Commission Division of Business Development, Government, and External Relations
Colette Bukowski, MA, LPCC-S, Associate Director, Business Development, Behavioral Health Care and Human Services; Julia S. Finken, BSN, MBA, CPHQ, CLSSMBB, Executive Director, Behavioral Health Care and Human Services

Joint Commission Division of Healthcare Improvement
Gina Malfeo-Martin, MSN, RN-BC, Associate Director, Standards Interpretation Group; Falguni Shah, MEd, LCPC, NCC, CHCEF, Associate Director, Clinical, Standards Interpretation Group

Joint Commission Division of Healthcare Quality Evaluation
Stacy Paul, MSN, RN, APN/PMHNP-BC, Project Director-Clinical, Standards and Survey Methods; Scott Williams, PsyD, Director of Research

Joint Commission Resources
Suzanne D, Harrison, MPH, Joint Commission Resources Continuous Service Readiness (CSR) Consultant/ Behavioral Health Specialist

Table of Contents

Introduction 5

Chapter 1: Screening for the Individualized Plan of Care 9

Introduction 11
The Preliminary Plan of Care 12
Identifying Individualized Needs, Strengths, Preferences, and Goals Through Screening 12
- Screening vs. Assessment 12
- Screening to Drive Decisions in Care 14
- Screening for Coordinated Care 15
- Screening for Suicide Risk 15

Additional Screening Challenges to Consider 20
- Some Contributing Factors 20
- Screening for Trauma 21
  - Successful Strategies: Integrating Trauma-Informed Care into Treatment Planning 21

Summary 23

Tool
- Tool 1-1. Sample Plan for Care Development Policy Template 24

Chapter 2: The Role of Assessment in the Individualized Plan 35

Introduction 36
Prioritizing Needs for Assessment 37
Importance of Reassessment 38
Using Assessment and Reassessment Tools 39
Evaluating Assessment Strategies 39
- Successful Strategies: Evaluating Your Assessment Forms 40

Including Identified Goals and Measurable Objectives 41
Common Challenges with Goals and Objectives 41
- Successful Strategies: Motivational Interviewing for Collaborative Goal Setting 42

Collaborative and Interdisciplinary Treatment Plans 42
Reevaluating and Revising Plan Goals and Objectives 43
- Challenges When Revising Plan Goals and Objectives 44
- Deferred Goals 44

Including Interventions That Meet Identified Goals 45
Involving Family in the Plan 46
Managing and Documenting a Referral 46
Summary 47

Tools
- Tool 2-1. Sample Patient Health Questionnaire-9 (PHQ-9) for Depression 48
- Tool 2-2. Sample Generalized Anxiety Disorder-7 (GAD-7) Questionnaire 49

Chapter 3: Integrating Measurement-Based Care in the Treatment Plan 51

Introduction 52
Criteria for Selecting a Measurement-Based Tool 53
Monitoring the Individual's Progress 54
Monitoring the Organization's Progress 55
Other Measurement-Based Instruments 55
Factors to Consider for Compliance 55
  Assessing Data Management 56
Using Data for Quality and Performance Improvement 56
Summary 57
Tools
  Tool 3-1. Sample Outcomes of Care, Treatment, or Services Measurement Procedures 58
  Tool 3-2. Sample Outcome Measurement Tracer Questions 62

Chapter 4: Planning for Unique Treatment Settings and Services 63

Introduction 66
Treatment Plans for Intensive Outpatient Programs 67
  Screening Considerations for Individuals with Addiction 67
  Assessment Considerations for Individuals with Addiction 68
  Building Individualized Treatment Plans for Individuals with Addiction 68
    Common Goals for Treatment 69
    Routine Testing and Monitoring 69
    Determining the Next Level of Service 70
Case Plans for Child Welfare Agencies 70
  A Trauma-Informed Case Plan 70
  Screening and Assessment Tools for Child Welfare 71
  Staff Requirements 71
  The Permanency Goal 71
  Assessing for Permanency 72
  After-Care Planning 73
Summary 73
Tool
  4-1. Standard Comprehensive Child and Adolescent Needs and Strengths (CANS) 3.0 Rating Sheet 75

Chapter 5: Sample Cases and Treatment Plans 83

Case #1: Ralph J. 83
  Sample Treatment Plan for Ralph J. 84
Case #2: Sheryl B. 88
  Sample Treatment Plan for Sheryl B. 89
Developing the Written Treatment Plan 89
Evaluating the Treatment Plan for Improvement 89
Summary 90
Tools
  5-1. Plan for Care, Treatment, or Services Template 91
  5-2. Plan for Care Evaluation Checklist 100

Glossary 103

Index 107

Introduction

Organizations that provide behavioral health care and human services (BHC) understand that millions of people in the United States are affected by behavioral health issues. According to the National Alliance on Mental Illness, in 2020, 46.2% of US adults with mental illness received treatment for various disorders,[1] and the World Health Organization reports that depression is a leading cause of disability worldwide and a major contributor to the overall global burden of disease.[2] Particularly now, with the COVID-19 pandemic, the demand for behavioral health care has never been higher. BHC organizations are increasingly challenged to provide the highest-quality treatment, care, and services. And that starts with **planning**. The Joint Commission understands the importance of screening and assessing individuals to ensure that the best care, treatment, or services are identified, planned, and then provided to those individuals. That is why The Joint Commission wrote this book. We want to help those individuals needing behavioral health care, treatment, or services. And we want to help our accredited BHC organizations understand how to successfully meet their needs.

When planning treatment, care, or services for individuals served, BHC organizations should consider four major dimensions of support for a life in recovery from behavioral health issues. Recovery—a process of change through which people improve their health and wellness, live directed lives, and strive to reach their full potential—requires the following[3]:

- Health: Overcoming or managing one's disease, disorder, or symptoms (for example, abstaining from alcohol, illicit drugs, or nonprescribed medications if one has an addiction problem) and making informed healthy choices that support physical and emotional well-being
- Home: Having a stable and safe place to live
- Purpose: Engaging in meaningful daily activities—such as work, school, volunteering, and creative activities—and having the independence and income to participate in society
- Community: Having relationships and social networks that provide support, friendship, love, and hope

About This Book

This book takes a close look at the Joint Commission standards and elements of performance (EPs) related to treatment planning in the "Care, Treatment, and Services" (CTS) chapter of the *Comprehensive Accreditation Manual for Behavioral Health Care and Human Services* (*CAMBHC*) and its counterpart E-dition®. It explores the processes and activities that go into effective treatment planning within BHC programs and settings. Of course, this book cannot delve into specific diagnoses and individual behavioral health care needs and planning for the appropriate treatment, care, or services to meet those needs. Rather, this book, like the Joint Commission standards, focuses on the quality of overall treatment planning processes within BHC organizations.

To help accredited BHC organizations identify and improve compliance in areas related to treatment planning, *Treatment Planning in Behavioral Health Care and Human Services* highlights Joint Commission requirements that many organizations find challenging (as seen by Joint Commission surveyors) and offers solutions and strategies for improvement. Recent data from The Joint Commission show that on surveys conducted in BHC settings in 2020, the rate of noncompliance with Standard CTS.03.01.03 was 61.69%. This requirement states: "The organization has a plan for care, treatment, or services that reflects the assessed needs, strengths, preferences, and goals of the individual served." That means that nearly two out of three Joint Commission–accredited BHC organizations surveyed in 2020 did not adequately plan for individuals' care, treatment, or services. What were the problems with complying with this requirement? Joint Commission surveyors reported the following common problems:

- Care, treatment, or service goals did not reflect the individual's own words.

- Care, treatment, or service goals were not reviewed at specific time frames as required.
- Care, treatment, or service goals were not measurable and did not or could not show progress toward meeting identified goals.
- The treatment plan did not address all the needs and problems identified during screening and assessment.
- The treatment plan was not individualized.
- Goals and objectives in multiple plans for multiple individuals were the same, selected from scripted language found in the electronic medical record.
- Individuals were not involved in decision making for treatment planning.
- Organizations failed to follow the written plan for care, treatment, or services.

This book will look at these compliance challenges and identify and explain ways that organizations can improve. Specifically, Joint Commission standards require BHC organizations to provide care, treatment, and services through the successful coordination and completion of the following processes:

- Entry to care, treatment, or services
- Screening, assessment, and reassessment
- Planning and development of care, treatment, or services
- Delivery of individualized care, treatment, or services
- Monitoring outcomes of care, treatment, or services to achieve individualized goals
- Continuity of care, treatment, or services
- Discharge planning
- Prevention and wellness promotion services, when applicable

This book will focus on these processes and activities to ensure that BHC organizations understand what is expected of them and how to comply. Not only did survey noncompliance data show the need for this book, in fact, BHC accredited organizations themselves asked for a book on this topic. Treatment planning in BHC was the #1 identified need on a survey conducted by Joint Commission Resources (JCR), The Joint Commission's official publisher and educator. Guidance on BHC treatment planning was also requested repeatedly at JCR's annual national BHC conference for accredited organizations.

Content Addressed in This Book

Treatment Planning in Behavioral Health Care and Human Services is divided into the following areas of focus:

- **Chapter 1: Screening for the Individualized Plan of Care.** This chapter focuses on screening, which lays the foundation for creating an effective individualized treatment plan. The key components of screening that inform an individualized plan of care for BHC organizations are addressed, including the following:
    - Identifying the needs, strengths, preferences, and goals of the individual through screening that helps drive decisions in care
    - Ensuring that the plan is individualized, and the individual served participates in decision making
    - Screening for suicide risk
    - Screening for trauma

- **Chapter 2: The Role of Assessment in the Individualized Plan.** This chapter explores the role of assessment and reassessment of the individual served to help confirm the presence of problems identified during screening, their scope and severity, and treatment options for addressing those problems. Topics addressed include the following:

SIDEBAR I-1 Although this book briefly addresses treatment planning for specific populations and programs, such as intensive outpatient programs and child welfare services, it does not attempt to provide guidance on treatment planning for all specialized populations and services. For example, programs accredited under The Joint Commission's Behavioral Health Home option and opioid treatment programs will not be addressed in detail in this book. Instead, guidance is provided for many of the standards that apply to all populations and programs within community BHC settings. Organizations accredited under such specialized programs and settings, such as the behavioral health home option or opioid addiction, should refer to the "Standards Applicability Process" (SAP) chapter of the *CAMBHC*, which helps those organizations determine which requirements and elements of performance apply directly to their setting(s), services, programs, and specific population(s).

- Ensuring that goals are expressed in the individual's own words or ideas
  - Ensuring that the plan includes measurable objectives informed by identified goals
  - Ensuring that goals are monitored, reevaluated, and revised when changes occur
  - Ensuring that the plan includes interventions and services required to meet identified goals and objectives
  - Identifying frequency of interventions and services and a time frame for review of goals and progress
  - Involving family, as appropriate
  - Ensuring an interdisciplinary and collaborative process when multiple disciplines are involved
  - Noting requirements for referrals and deferrals (in other words, what an organization should do when it cannot meet the needs of the individual)

- **Chapter 3: Integrating Measurement-Based Care in the Treatment Plan.** This chapter outlines the steps organizations can take to improve outcomes by integrating measurement-based care, tools, and instruments in treatment planning. It includes guidance on standardized monitoring, evaluating the effectiveness of treatment plans, and aggregating data for improvements in care for individuals served as well as for the organization.

- **Chapter 4: Planning for Unique Treatment Settings and Services.** This chapter addresses some of the more unique treatment planning requirements for organizations providing care, treatment, and services for individuals seeking addiction services and for child welfare agencies. These settings are by no means representative of all specialized populations or service settings but are used only to illustrate some unique planning activities for these settings and services. In 2020 The Joint Commission released new and revised requirements for BHC organizations that treat substance use disorders. These requirements aim to improve successful transitions of care and follow-up and proper drug testing as components of treatment planning in this setting. Also in 2020 The Joint Commission added and revised expectations for development and review of case plans for child welfare agencies. Changes in this area aim to improve child welfare for individuals and families served by adoption agencies, foster care, and child protective services, to name a few. This chapter briefly looks at some unique requirements that go beyond what is required for all BHC organizations.

- **Chapter 5: Sample Cases and Treatment Plans.** This chapter offers two typical scenarios that BHC organizations might encounter and includes sample treatment plans for these scenarios. In addition, this chapter includes tools that will help practitioners develop their own written treatment plans and evaluate them for continued compliance.

In addition, select chapters include the following:

- Relevant Joint Commission standards and EPs: A list of key standards and EPs are included that correspond to the main topics addressed.
  Note: Joint Commission standards are updated on a regular basis. Always refer to the most current version of the *CAMBHC* or its E-dition counterpart for requirements relevant to your setting. The standards in this book are those in effect at the time of publication.
- Terms to Know: Key terms and concepts are called out in each chapter and defined in a Glossary to help with understanding.
- Tools to Use: Included in each chapter are forms, checklists, and templates to assist BHC professionals with screening, assessment, planning, and evaluation to create more effective treatment and case plans.

Audience for This Book

This book was developed for anyone in a BHC organization who needs to understand The Joint Commission's requirements for treatment planning—in particular, Joint Commission accreditation professionals who are responsible for ensuring their organizations' compliance and BHC professionals who are responsible for actually creating treatment and case plans. Those responsible for risk management and performance improvement in BHC organizations will also benefit from this book. Finally, this book will assist nonaccredited BHC organizations looking for best practices in treatment planning.

Acknowledgments

JCR acknowledges the time and insight of all reviewers at The Joint Commission. We thank and recognize Jennifer Johnson, MEd, MBA, LPC, Joint Commission Behavioral Health Care and Human Services Surveyor, for her role as editor; Suzanne D. Harrison, MPH, Joint Commission Resources Continuous Service Readiness (CSR) Consultant/Behavioral Health Specialist for contributing the case scenarios in Chapter 5; and writer Mollie Page for her assistance in pulling it all together.

Tools to Use

The tools in this book are available as downloadable, customizable resources that can be distributed internally to health care staff. To access these tools, click on **DOWNLOAD** the complete tool icon, or visit https://store-jcrinc.ae-admin.com/assets/1/7/TPBH21_Landing_Page.pdf

References

1. National Alliance on Mental Illness. Mental Health by the Numbers. (Updated: Mar 2021.) Accessed Dec 21, 2021. https://www.nami.org/mhstats.
2. World Health Organization. Depression. Sep 13, 2021. Accessed Dec 21, 2021. https://www.who.int/en/news-room/fact-sheets/detail/depression.
3. Substance Abuse and Mental Health Services Administration. Recovery and Recovery Support. (Updated: Apr 23, 2020.) Accessed Dec 21, 2021. https://www.samhsa.gov/find-help/recovery

Chapter 1
Screening for the Individualized Plan of Care

Relevant Standards Covered in This Chapter	
CTS.01.03.01	The organization develops a preliminary plan for care, treatment, or services, when needed. **Note:** For child welfare agencies, this plan might include a safety plan.
	EP 1 The organization develops a preliminary plan for care, treatment, or services when care, treatment, or services are initiated prior to completion of the screening and assessment process.
	EP 2 The preliminary plan for care, treatment, or services focuses on the individual's safety and addresses interventions in response to emergency needs, such as an immediate need for placement or danger to self or others.
CTS.02.01.01	The organization has a screening procedure for the early detection of risk of imminent harm to self or others.
	EP 1 The screening procedure determines the need for immediate intervention to protect the individual served or others.
	EP 2 The organization follows its process for responding when an immediate risk of harm to self or others is identified. **Note:** The process may include referring the individual to another organization.
CTS.02.01.09	The organization screens all individuals served for physical pain.
CTS.02.01.11	The organization screens all individuals served for their nutritional status.
	EP 1 The organization screens all individuals served to identify those for whom a nutritional assessment is indicated. At a minimum, the screening includes questions about the following: • Food allergies • Weight loss or gain of 10 pounds or more in the last 3 months • Decrease in food intake and/or appetite • Dental problems • Eating habits or behaviors that may be indicators of an eating disorder, such as bingeing or induced vomiting
CTS.02.02.05	The organization identifies individuals who may have experienced trauma, abuse, neglect, or exploitation.
	EP 1 The organization educates staff about trauma, abuse, neglects, and exploitation and how to refer individuals, as needed. Note: Staff should be able to screen for trauma, abuse, neglect, and exploitation as indicated by the needs or conditions of the individual served. The organization may define who conducts the assessment for alleged or suspected trauma, abuse, neglect, and exploitation or when to refer to another organization.

Relevant Standards Covered in This Chapter	
	EP 2 The organization identifies individuals who may have experienced trauma, abuse, neglect, or exploitation during initial screening and on an ongoing basis. **Note:** For child welfare: The agency also defines family members, including from the family of origin and/or resource family, who may have experienced trauma, abuse, neglect, or exploitation. The agency defines which family members to include in this process.
CTS.03.01.01	The organization bases the planned care, treatment, or services on the needs, strengths, preferences, and goals of the individual served.
	EP 1 In collaboration with the individual served and, as appropriate, their family, the organization makes care, treatment, or service decisions that are based on information it has collected about the individual's needs, strengths, preferences, and goals.
	EP 2 Care, treatment, or service decisions are collaborative and interdisciplinary when more than one discipline is involved in the care, treatment, or services of the individual served.
	EP 4 Planning for care, treatment, or services includes interventions and services necessary to meet the identified goals.
NPSG.15.01.01	Reduce the risk for suicide.
	EP 1 The organization conducts an environmental risk assessment that identifies features in the physical environment that could be used to attempt suicide and takes necessary action to minimize the risk(s) (for example, removal of anchor points, door hinges, and hooks that can be used for hanging). **Note:** Noninpatient behavioral health care and human services settings and unlocked inpatient units do not need to be ligature resistant. The expectation for these settings is to conduct a risk assessment to identify potential environmental hazards to individuals served, identify individuals who are at high risk for suicide, and take action to safeguard these individuals from the environmental risks (for example, continuous monitoring in a safe location while awaiting transfer to higher level of care and removing objects from the room that can be used for self-harm).
	EP 2 Screen all individuals served for suicidal ideation using a validated screening tool. **Note:** The Joint Commission requires screening for suicidal ideation using a validated tool starting at age 12 and above.
	EP 3 Use an evidence-based process to conduct a suicide assessment of individuals served who have screened positive for suicidal ideation. The assessment directly asks about suicidal ideation, plan, intent, suicidal or self-harm behaviors, risk factors, and protective factors. **Note:** EPs 2 and 3 can be satisfied through the use of a single process or instrument that simultaneously screens individuals served for suicidal ideation and assesses the severity of suicidal ideation.
	EP 4 Document individuals' overall level of risk for suicide and the plan to mitigate the risk for suicide.
	EP 5 Follow written policies and procedures addressing the care of individuals served identified as at risk for suicide. At a minimum, these should include the following: • Training and competence assessment of staff who care for individuals served at risk for suicide • Guidelines for reassessment • Monitoring individuals served who are at high risk for suicide
	EP 6 Follow written policies and procedures for counseling and follow-up care at discharge for individuals served identified as at risk for suicide.
	EP 7 Monitor implementation and effectiveness of policies and procedures for screening, assessment, and management of individuals served at risk for suicide and take action as needed to improve compliance.

Note: Joint Commission standards are updated on a regular basis. Always refer to the most current version of the *Comprehensive Accreditation Manual for Behavioral Health Care and Human Services* (*CAMBHC*) or its E-dition® counterpart for requirements relevant to your setting.

Terms to Know

assessment
goals
needs
treatment plan, or plan of care, treatment, or services
preferences
scope of service
screening
strengths
trauma

Introduction

This chapter focuses on the Joint Commission requirements that inform an *individualized* plan of care, treatment, or services, or treatment plan, in behavioral health care and human services (BHC) settings and explores key processes for developing an effective treatment plan, including the following:

- Creating the preliminary plan of care
- Identifying the needs, strengths, preferences, and goals of the individual through screening and assessment
- Ensuring that the plan is individualized, that the individual participates in decision making, and that the same "scripted" language is not used for all individuals served
- Ensuring that goals include the individual's own words and express the individual's ideas
- Ensuring that the plan includes measurable, identified goals and objectives
- Ensuring that goals are monitored, reevaluated, and revised, and outcomes are measured as individuals progress through treatment
- Ensuring that the plan includes interventions and services required to meet identified goals and objectives
- Including the frequency of interventions, services, and a time frame for reviewing goals and progress
- Incorporating family involvement into the treatment or case plan, as appropriate
- Ensuring that the plan is interdisciplinary and collaborative when multiple disciplines are involved
- Addressing referrals, particularly what an organization should do when it cannot meet the needs of the individual served

A **treatment plan**, or plan of care, treatment, or services, simply stated, is a written plan, based on data gathered during screening and assessment, that identifies care, treatment, or service needs, strengths, preferences, and goals; describes the strategy for meeting those needs, preferences, and goals; builds on the strengths and considers the preferences of the individuals served; and documents progress toward meeting the plan's objectives. The plan may include care, treatment, habilitation, and rehabilitation.

To build an effective treatment plan, and to comply with Joint Commission requirements, organizations must coordinate the care, treatment, and services they provide in a manner that is consistent with their **scope of service**. The organization's scope of service is the activities defined by the organization and permitted by relevant licensing authorities as descriptive of the services the organization provides. It helps define the organization's capabilities based on its resources and expertise. When crafting admission and exclusionary criteria, the organization's scope of service informs creation of a treatment plan.

A sample plan of care development policy template (Tool 1-1 on page 24) can help guide organizations to develop a policy for creating individualized plans for care. The template addresses the important steps for creating a Joint Commission–compliant treatment plan including staff responsibilities, plan development, and plan review. The template includes an overview of procedures for specific settings accredited under the BHC program and can be modified as appropriate for an organization's services. When establishing policies and procedures for treatment plan development, it is critical that organizations consider the following:

- All care, treatment, or services provided
- All active care, treatment, and services received elsewhere and relevant information from those treatment providers
- Coordination of care with internal and external providers
- All areas of the organization that participate in the care, treatment, or services of individuals served
- All staff members who participate in the care, treatment, or services of individuals served
- All individuals who can receive care, treatment, or services from the organization

The screening processes discussed in this chapter are meant to provide a foundation for developing treatment plans that ensure high-quality, focused, individualized care. Such care may include symptom management, timely delivery of support, clinical direction, and guidance for targeted therapies and interventions that emphasize the individualization and specificity of the treatment plan.

The Preliminary Plan of Care

Frequently misunderstood, The Joint Commission's Care, Treatment, and Services (CTS) Standard CTS.01.03.01, related to the preliminary plan of care, requires accredited organizations to develop a preliminary plan of care, ***when needed***, prior to completion of screening and assessment processes. The rationale for this requirement is to address the safety needs of the individual served.

A preliminary plan, for example, would be needed for a behavioral health emergency, which is a life-threatening situation in which an individual in danger of harm to self or to others, is severely disoriented or out of touch with reality, or is otherwise out of control. A child welfare agency may consider a preliminary plan of care for a minor at risk of neglect, domestic violence, sexual exploitation, elopement, or sexually reactive behaviors stemming from a report from a state-mandated reporter, such as a teacher or licensed caregiver.

A preliminary treatment plan starts the treatment process and stems from initial interview, intake information, and evaluation of that information. The goal of the preliminary plan of care is to identify and address the individual's immediate needs. Many BHC organizations allow for a time frame (for example 72 hours) for completion of screening and assessment by all clinical disciplines involved in an individual's care to create a comprehensive treatment plan. However, if the individual has emergency needs that must be addressed immediately, such as a minor in an abusive home who needs a safe place to stay, then actual treatment or services may need to begin before a fully formed treatment plan is developed. A preliminary plan of care provides a guiding conceptualization of those immediate services needed, the goals and objectives underlying the provision of services, and who is responsible for providing those services.

A preliminary plan of care focuses on addressing interventions in response to the emergency need (a safe place to stay) and provides structure and framework for initiating treatment that, at minimum, addresses an individual's safety. The preliminary plan of care may start the treatment process of working toward a more comprehensive document that identifies care, treatment, or service needs, as well as strengths, preferences, and goals; describes the strategy for meeting those needs, preferences, and goals; builds on the strengths and considers the preferences of the individuals served; and documents progress toward meeting the plan's objectives.

Identifying Individualized Needs, Strengths, Preferences, and Goals Through Screening

The first step in developing a comprehensive treatment plan is to identify the needs, strengths, preferences, and goals of the individual served. This is done first through screening, which we will address in detail below, and assessment, which is discussed in detail in Chapter 2, by qualified staff.

Screening vs. Assessment

The terms ***screening*** and ***assessment*** are sometimes used interchangeably, but there are key differences between the two activities. Screening can indicate a need for assessment. The main purpose of screening is to provide a high-level check on the presence of risk factors that could indicate a problem. Screening is typically done by trained and qualified intake staff, which may include clinicians or support staff. It happens at admission or during an initial encounter with an individual and is generally brief, with a narrow scope.

Assessment delves deeper into an individual's risk factors to get a more comprehensive clinical picture of the individual. Its purpose is to aid in the diagnosis and/or treatment planning for the individual, by identifying conditions and their severity to inform treatment recommendations. Assessment incorporates information from multiple, in-depth sources, including screenings. Assessment is generally completed in accordance with a time frame defined by the organization or required by state law or regulation.

Together screening and assessment identify the type and level of care, treatment, or services by considering the individual's needs, strengths, preferences, and goals. Key to both are data collection and analysis as well as documentation to record and support planning, delivery, and continuity of care, treatment, or services. Screening and assessment have a sequential relationship—screening typically comes first and may or may not trigger assessment, depending on the outcome of the screening process. Staff who perform these processes must be competent to perform the tasks and duties of their job description and determined by the scope of an organization's practice, state law, and/or regulations.

For example, as part of an organization's intake screening practices, an individual seeking treatment for depression may reveal recent and excessive weight gain and that he hasn't had a physical health examination in five years. Based on this screening data, and as part of its assessment practices, the organization might then administer a diagnostic, evidence-based tool to measure the severity of the individual's depression and might also perform a physical exam—or refer the individual for a physical exam—to assess the individual's physical health status. In another example, an individual referred for follow-up care after treatment for a suicide attempt screens positive for suicide risk at intake but does not currently have suicidal thoughts. Further assessment is still required, including the individual's history of suicidal ideation, self-harm behaviors, risk factors, and protective factors to determine that individual's overall risk for suicide. This aligns with Joint Commission requirements for reducing suicide risks. All such screening and assessment data are analyzed and used to drive appropriate individualized care.

The Joint Commission requires screening individuals for the following:

- Physical health (CTS.02.01.05 through CTS.02.01.07), including processes for identifying individuals' medical history and the need for a physical examination
- Physical pain (CTS.02.01.09), including screening for the presence, duration, and acuity of any physical pain
- Nutritional status (CTS.02.01.11), such as food allergies, recent significant weight loss or gain, decrease in food intake and/or appetite
- Trauma, abuse (which can be physical, sexual, emotional, financial, and so on), neglect, and exploitation (CTS.02.02.05)
- Specific screening and assessment for identified populations, settings, or services, such as addiction, individuals with intellectual and development disorders, child welfare, eating disorders, and so on*
- Screening for harm to self or others (CTS.02.01.01), including screening for self-injury and violent/homicidal behaviors
- Suicide risk (National Patient Safety Goal [NPSG] Standard NPSG.15.01.01), requires use of a validated screening tool and an evidence-based process to identify level of risk for suicide.

An individual's **needs** are the basic necessities required to produce a good treatment outcome as identified during screening, but it is important to note that needs may change and new needs may arise that need to be prioritized throughout the course of treatment. For example, an individual arrested for driving under the influence of alcohol may be mandated by law to receive substance use treatment. That person's primary need is treatment for substance use. However, during the course of treatment for alcohol use, a new need arises when the individual expresses a need to rebuild a failed relationship with her adult son. Her treatment will prioritize meeting her legal requirement. In addition, the work required to improve her relationship with her son may not be feasibly accomplished during the time frame the organization has to work with her. However, it may be possible to address the work required to repair the failed relationship for a later time to help ensure a better treatment outcome for the individual served. When planning treatment, BHC organizations must put the individual's expressed needs into the context of what can realistically be addressed given its particular level of care, its programs/services, and the amount of time it has to work with the individual.

Factors that support the health and well-being of an individual and empower that individual with positive purpose, are considered the individual's **strengths**.

* Refer to the *Comprehensive Accreditation Manual for Behavioral Health Care and Human Services* (*CAMBHC*) or corresponding E-dition® for detailed screening and assessment standards for specific populations and programs.

Included among individuals' strengths are such things as religious beliefs or faith, support network of family and/or friends, ability to work or care for others, and capacity for hope. When screening adults, questions that address friends, work, spouses or children, life experiences, or hobbies can help identify strengths such as the following:

- Tell me about the strengths and resources you've used in the past to remain sober.
- Some people have others in their life who support them or model successful behavior. Who do you have in your life who does that for you?
- Tell me about your achievements at work, with friends, in sports, with family, or in past treatment.

Individuals' strengths can help in the development of objectives and interventions in their plan. For example, an individual who has expressed being good with numbers and liking detailed work, may establish a short-term objective of volunteering at a local library as a pathway to full-time employment and independent living. Developing objectives and interventions for the treatment plan will be addressed in more detail in Chapter 2.

An individual's personal **preferences** will largely account for whether that individual will be actively engaged in treatment and involve such things as preference for appointment time, communication format (in-person or virtual), language proficiency, adherence to cultural norms or beliefs, spirituality, and so on. Cultural beliefs, for example, may have a strong influence on the individual served and on the attitudes of the family members and support networks of that individual. For example, a middle-aged woman who has been in treatment for depression since her divorce two years ago, continues to feel guilt and shame about her divorce. She was raised to believe divorce was unacceptable and has been ostracized by her family. Intellectually she knows the divorce was the best decision for her, and she is sad and angry with her family for judging her. The influence of the attitude of her family and the lack of their support may be a barrier to a successful treatment outcome.

Simply stated, **goals** are the achievable outcomes for care, treatment, or services. However, in treatment planning, The Joint Commission requires that goals be expressed by the individual served, identified in clear language, built on the strengths of the individual, and include measurable, time-bound objectives. Goals may be long term (for example, "I want to have an apartment on my own someday"), or they may be short term, such as "I want to make an appointment with a doctor for a physical." In Chapter 2 we will discuss how to incorporate individualized goals in the treatment plan.

Screening to Drive Decisions in Care

Your organization's policies and procedures dictate what information is to be collected from individuals served, family/guardian, or others as permitted by the individual and other providers. This is driven primarily by your organization's scope of service. It may also be determined by the individual's emergent needs or the care, treatment, or services that individual is seeking. For example, if after screening it is determined that an individual has a substance use disorder and this is beyond the organization's scope of service, the organization may provide resources or refer the individual to another provider.

In some cases, such as when treating individuals with intellectual and developmental disability (IDD) or for child welfare agencies, it may be necessary to rely on other sources because the primary individual served has limited ability to provide the information. However, this is not exclusive to these settings. Practitioners may be required to collect collateral information, if appropriate and available, from an individual's family member or guardian to provide appropriate care. Effective and thorough data collection through screening processes is a key part of a holistic approach to getting to know the individual served. Accurately identifying the needs of the individual served, incorporating those needs into the written plan, and modifying the plan in accordance with progress toward goals and changes in needs are the basis for high-quality care.

Organizations can improve compliance in their screening processes by examining how their screening is performed, what information is gathered and by whom, and when screening takes place. For example, screening that relies solely on data collected from a standard self-report biopsychosocial form—a form used by organizations to capture biological, psychological, and social data from an individual—that an individual completes alone in a reception room may not capture a complete picture of that individual's needs. Individuals' current emotional or behavioral state may prevent them from being forthcoming about past behaviors or treatment in this environment. Individuals who, by virtue of their mental health condition, are unable to participate in screening, as well as those individuals who are not voluntarily seeking care, treatment, or services, present considerable challenges to the BHC organization. In these cases, past medical records and/or diagnoses and input from family members, for example, may prove to be a useful part of screening practices.

Screening for Coordinated Care

Individuals with serious mental illness and chronic medical conditions (for example, diabetes, hypertension) die 20 to 25 years earlier than those who do not have chronic medical conditions. And because of their mental illness, these individuals are often not as aware of or tend to their physical health as much as those who do not have serious mental illness.[1] As a result, it is critical for BHC organizations to screen all individuals served for physical health, pain, and nutrition and to complete further assessments, as needed.

In some BHC settings, The Joint Commission requires organizations to determine whether the date of the individual's most current physical exam exceeds one year. If the date exceeds one year, then a medical history and physical examination must be performed. If performing a medical history and physical exam is outside the organization's scope of service, it may refer the individual to another organization. Organizations must have a process for securing the individual's agreement to receive a medical history and physical exam, which should be included in the individual's treatment plan of care.

The Joint Commission also requires BHC organizations to ensure that staff who perform screening are competent in their duties and trained in their organization's policies and procedures, which are determined by scope of service and state laws and/or regulations.

A regular review of your organization's screening practices may include evaluation of your facility's screening tools, practices, and procedures. For example, does the organization's policy include a practice for appropriate and timely follow-up on screening results? When auditing treatment plans, are issues identified during the course of treatment that were missed during screening? Are staff qualified, trained, and competent in screening processes? Are screening tools and forms current and inclusive; for example, in terms of gender language?

Screening for Suicide Risk

According to the Centers for Disease Control and Prevention (CDC) the prevalence of suicidal ideation doubled among respondents during the COVID-19 pandemic as compared to rates of surveyed adults in 2018.[2] As part of its National Patient Safety Goals, The Joint Commission's Standard NPSG.15.01.01 requires BHC organizations to screen for suicide risk using a validated screening tool for all individuals starting at age 12 and above. For individuals under the age of 12, the organization determines if, when, and how to screen for suicide.

Yet, screening for suicidal ideation continues to challenge many organizations. In fact, among surveys conducted in 2020 for the BHC program setting, 40% of organizations were found noncompliant with NPSG.15.01.01, particularly the requirements for using a validated screening tool, orienting and training staff on the proper use of the tool selected, and following the organization's written policies and procedures when addressing the care of individuals who screened positive for suicide ideation. Surveyor observations cited staff training and competence as particularly challenging areas.

Other issues include, for example, not knowing how to respond when an individual refuses to participate in screening and using "informal" screening, such as simply asking a few questions about suicidal ideation, as opposed to using a validated tool to ensure standardization and reliability across staff, which is required by The Joint Commission.

NPSG.15.01.01 requires BHC organizations to not only screen for suicide risk but also to identify the overall level of risk by using an evidence-based assessment process. If the validated screening tool used by a facility indicates that an individual is at risk for suicide, that individual will need an evidenced-based suicide risk assessment to determine next steps.

Based on level of risk, organizations must determine the most appropriate mitigation strategies and whether transfer to a different level of care is warranted. In addition, an environmental risk assessment must be conducted by the organization to identify anything that could be used to attempt suicide. It is important to document any actions taken to minimize risk(s) for suicide, such as removing physical items that could be used to attempt suicide, including blinds with pull cords, scissors, or trash bags, for example. However, it is also important to note that noninpatient settings and unlocked inpatient units are not required by The Joint Commission to be ligature resistant. The expectation is for the organizations to identify environmental hazards to the individual served, identify individuals who are at high risk for suicide, and take actions to ensure that those individuals are safe from environmental risk (for example, through continuous monitoring in a safe location that is free from objects that can be used for self-harm, until the high-risk individual can be transferred to a higher level of care).

The Joint Commission requires that when organizations screen individuals for risk of suicide, screening incorporates the following:

- Use of a validated tool (*see* Table 1-1 for a list of validated suicide prevention screening tools and resources). Keep in mind that this list is not exhaustive, and The Joint Commission does not prescribe the use of any one particular tool.
- Provision for input from parent, guardian, or significant other, as appropriate
- Evidence-based processes to assess individuals who have screened positive for suicidal ideation

For compliance, organizations must have a process in place to monitor the effectiveness of their suicide prevention program and ensure that their screening tools meet requirements, including appropriateness for the individuals served.

Table 1-1. Examples of Validated, Evidence-Based Suicide Prevention Screening Tools

This compendium of suicide prevention screening resources includes validated, evidence-based tools that can be used when screening for suicide risk. The Joint Commission does not prescribe the use of any particular tool included in this list, and this list is not exhaustive. Organizations must choose suicide prevention screening tools that are appropriate to the individuals they serve.

Tools	Brief Description
Ask Suicide-Screening Questions (ASQ) Toolkit by the National Institute of Mental Health (NIMH) **Authors:** NIMH **Settings:** Emergency departments, medical/surgical unit, outpatient primary care, specialty clinics **Population:** All ages **Availability:** Free: **www.nimh.nih.gov/asq**	The **Ask Suicide-Screening Questions (ASQ)** toolkit was developed and validated by a team from the National Institute for Mental Health (NIMH) following a 2008 multisite study. ASQ is a four-item suicide-screening tool designed to be used for people of all ages in emergency departments, inpatient units, and primary care facilities. A Brief Suicide Safety Assessment (BSSA) is available to be used when patients screen positive for suicide risk on the ASQ. The toolkit is organized by the medical setting in which it will be used: emergency department, inpatient medical/surgical unit, and outpatient primary care and specialty clinics. The ASQ is free of charge and available in multiple languages. All toolkit materials are available on the NIMH website at **www.nimh.nih.gov/asq**.

(continued)

Tools	Brief Description
	Recommending Organizations: 1. National Institute for Mental Health (NIMH) 2. National Action Alliance for Suicide Prevention (Action Alliance): Transforming Health Systems Initiative Work Group. *Recommended Standard Care for People with Suicide Risk: Making Health Care Suicide Safe*. Washington, DC: Education Development Center, Inc., 2018. 3. Zero Suicide Initiative: **http://zerosuicide.edc.org/** **Evidence/Development:** 1. Horowitz LM, et al. Ask Suicide-Screening Questions (ASQ): A brief instrument for the pediatric emergency department. *Arch Pediatr Adolesc Med*. 2012 Dec;166(12):1170–1176. doi: 10.1001/archpediatrics.2012.1276
Columbia-Suicide Severity Rating Scale (C-SSRS) Triage version **Authors:** Columbia University, the University of Pennsylvania, and the University of Pittsburgh—supported by the National Institute of Mental Health (NIMH) **Settings:** General, health care **Population:** All ages **Availability:** Free: **https://cssrs.columbia.edu/**	The **Columbia-Suicide Severity Rating Scale (C-SSRS)** evidence-supported screening tool was developed by Columbia University, the University of Pennsylvania, and the University of Pittsburgh, supported by the National Institute of Mental Health (NIMH). The C-SSRS Triage version features questions that help determine whether an individual is at risk for suicide. There are brief versions of the C-SSRS often used as a screening tool (first two questions) that, based on patient response, can lead to the administration of the additional questions to triage patients. The protocol and the training on how to use it are available free of charge. This **triage guide** shows how some different types of programs are using the worrisome answers to guide clinical decision making (for example, does the patient require 1:1 observation or a psychiatrist to consult?). The triage model embeds the Columbia Protocol into the electronic health record (EHR)/electronic medical record (EMR) and provides alerts for high-risk answers. There is no cost or license required for health/behavioral care providers to put the Columbia Protocol tools into the EHR/EMR. **Recommending Organizations:** 1. National Institutes of Health (NIH) 2. Substance Abuse and Mental Health Services Administration (SAMHSA) 3. National Action Alliance for Suicide Prevention (Action Alliance) 4. US Department of Defense 5. Centers for Disease Control and Prevention (CDC), National Center for Injury Prevention and Control 6. US Food and Drug Administration (FDA) 7. Zero Suicide Initiative: **https://zerosuicide.edc.org/** **Evidence/Development:** 1. The Columbia Lighthouse Project/Center for Suicide Risk Assessment. The Columbia Suicide Severity Rating Scale (C-SSRS) Supporting Evidence. Last revised Jan 14, 2020: **https://cssrs.columbia.edu/wp-content/uploads/CSSRS_Supporting-Evidence_Book_2020-01-14.pdf** 2. Posner K, et al. The Columbia–Suicide Severity Rating Scale: Initial validity and internal consistency findings from three multisite studies with adolescents and adults. *Am J Psychiatry*. 2011 Dec;168(12):1266–1277. doi: 10.1176/appi.ajp.2011.10111704

(continued)

Tools	Brief Description
Patient Health Questionnaire-9 (PHQ-9) Depression Scale **Authors:** Drs. Robert L. Spitzer, Janet B.W. Williams, Kurt Kroenke, and colleagues, with an educational grant from Pfizer Inc. **Settings:** Primary care, behavioral health care and human services (BHC) **Population:** Adults, age 12+ **Availability:** Free: **https://www.phqscreeners.com/select-screener** (All PHQ, GAD-7 [Generalized Anxiety Disorder scale] screeners and translations are downloadable from this website, and no permission is required to reproduce, translate, display, or distribute them).	The **Patient Health Questionnaire-9 (PHQ-9) Depression Scale** is a validated, widely used nine-item tool used to diagnose and monitor the severity of depression. Question 9 screens for the presence and duration of suicide ideation. It is available in Spanish and other languages and has also been modified for the adolescent population. All screening tools and instruction manuals are available at no cost: **https://www.phqscreeners.com/select-screener**. **Recommending Organizations:** 1. AIMS Center University of Washington 2. Substance Abuse and Mental Health Services Administration (SAMHSA) 3. National Action Alliance for Suicide Prevention (Action Alliance): Transforming Health Systems Initiative Work Group. *Recommended Standard Care for People with Suicide Risk: Making Health Care Suicide Safe*. Washington, DC: Education Development Center, Inc., 2018. 4. Zero Suicide Initiative: **https://zerosuicide.edc.org/** **Evidence:** 1. Simon GE, et al. Does response on the PHQ-9 depression questionnaire predict subsequent suicide attempt or suicide death? *Psychiatr Serv*. 2013 Dec;64(12):1195–1202. doi: 10.1176/appi.ps.201200587 2. Rossom RC, et al. Suicidal Ideation reported on the PHQ9 and risk of suicidal behavior across age groups. *J Affect Discord*. 2017 Jun;215:77–84. doi: 10.1016/j.jad.2017.03.037 3. Louzon SA, et al. Does suicidal ideation as measured by the PHQ-9 predict suicide among VA patients? *Psychiatr Serv*. 2016 May 1;67(5):517–522. doi: 10.1176/appi.ps.201500149
Suicide Behavior Questionnaire-Revised (SBQ-R, Osman et al., 2001) **Population:** ages 13–18	The **Suicide Behavior Questionnaire-Revised (SBQ-R)** is a four-item self-report questionnaire that asks about future anticipation of suicidal thoughts or behaviors, as well as past and present ones, and includes a question about lifetime suicidal ideation, plans to commit suicide, and actual attempts. Item 1 evaluates lifetime ideation and attempt, Item 2 assesses frequency of ideation in the past 12 months, Item 3 explores suicide threats, and Item 4 evaluates the likelihood of future suicidal behavior. **Recommending Organizations:** 1. National Action Alliance for Suicide Prevention (Action Alliance): Transforming Health Systems Initiative Work Group. Recommended Standard Care for People with Suicide Risk: Making Health Care Suicide Safe. Washington, DC: Education Development Center, Inc., 2018. **Evidence:** 1. Brown GK. *A Review of Suicide Assessment Measures for Intervention Research with Adults and Older Adults*. Bethesda, MD: National Institute of Mental Health, 2003. **https://www.sprc.org/resources-programs/review-suicide-assessment-measures-intervention-research-adults-older-adults** 2. Osman A, et al. The Suicidal Behaviors Questionnaire-Revised (SBQ-R): Validation with clinical and nonclinical samples. *Assessment*. 2001 Dec;8(4):443–454. doi: 10.1177/107319110100800409 3. Kreuze E, Lamis D. A review of psychometrically tested instruments assessing suicide risk in adults. *Omega* (Westport). 2018 May;77(1):36–90. doi: 10.1177/0030222816688151

(continued)

Tools	Brief Description
Suicide risk screening in pediatric hospitals: Clinical pathways to address a global health crisis **Authors:** Dr. Khyati Brahmbhatt and colleagues (*Psychosomatics*. 2019 Jan–Feb;60(1):1–9) **https://www.sciencedirect.com/science/article/pii/S0033318218304298**	This paper details the first interdisciplinary and international effort to generate clinical pathways (CPs) for pediatric suicide risk screening in general hospital settings. The clinical pathway was created as a guide for hospitals worldwide to improve youth suicide risk screening and implementation of appropriate next steps. The pathway includes the use of the Ask Suicide-Screening Questions (ASQ) (brief primary screener) and the Columbia-Suicide Severity Rating Scale (C-SSRS) or the ASQ Brief Suicide Safety Assessment (secondary screeners) for screening and risk stratification of suicidality in children and adolescents in medical settings (14–17). The publication includes four appendices: • The introductory document (Appendix A) is intended to help orient providers, managers, and administrators in a variety of disciplines and specialties to the pathway. • The flow diagrams (Appendix B: 1–3) visually depict the steps in the clinical pathways for suicide risk screening in the emergency department (Appendix B.1) and in the pediatric inpatient medical/surgical setting (Appendix B.2). Both pathways describe a similar three-tiered screening process. Further, a brief suicide risk screening for the C-SSRS was created for hospitals that may already be using this scale (Appendix B.3). • The text document (Appendix C) contains a narrative description of the pathway that is to be used side by side with the flow diagrams by individuals or institutions implementing a pediatric suicide risk screening process within their institution. • Sample scripts for conducting an ASQ screen, the Brief Suicide Safety Assessment, and steps taken after are provided in Appendix D.
Recommended Standard Care for People with Suicide Risk: Making Health Care Suicide Safe. Washington, DC: Education Development Center, Inc. **Author:** National Action Alliance for Suicide Prevention (Action Alliance): Transforming Health Systems Initiative Work Group (2018) **Settings:** Primary care, behavioral health, emergency departments **Availability:** Free: **https://theactionalliance.org/resource/recommended-standard-care**	The **Recommended Standard Care for People with Suicide Risk: Making Health Care Suicide Safe** report provides recommendations on suicide-related standard health care for primary care, behavioral health, and emergency department settings. It was produced by health care and suicide prevention experts working with the National Action Alliance for Suicide Prevention (Action Alliance). The information is intended to guide health care organizations that wish to better identify and support people who are at increased risk of suicide and for advocates who will work with hospitals and clinics to make them safer. The report describes why improving suicide care is urgently needed; identifies gaps in health care that contribute to suicide deaths; summarizes the evidence-based solutions that should be adopted; and provides information on resources that are available to make care safer and better.

(continued)

Tools	Brief Description
ED-SAFE Study Materials **The Patient Safety Screener (PSS-3): A Brief Tool to Detect Suicide Risk in Acute Care Settings** **Author:** Emergency Medicine Network (EMNet) **Settings:** Emergency departments **Availability:** Free: **http://www.sprc.org/micro-learnings/patientsafetyscreener**	ED-SAFE is an NIMH-funded, eight-site suicide prevention project. The major goals are to examine the impact of screening emergency department (ED) patients for suicide risk, the effect of an ED-initiated intervention on suicidal behavior, and the economic impacts of treatment as usual, screening, and the intervention. The ED-SAFE resource collection includes **provider guidance and training tools**, the **Patient Safety Screener** to be administered by ED nursing staff, and **Patient Safety Secondary Screener** to assess if referral to mental health treatment is warranted. Resources also include **patient handouts** in English and Spanish for self-care, how to stay safe, and a personal safety plan.

Source: Suicide Prevention Resources to support Joint Commission Accredited Organizations Implementation of NPSG 15.01.01, revised July 2020. Accessed Dec 21, 2021. **https://www.jointcommission.org/-/media/tjc/documents/resources/patient-safety-topics/suicide-prevention/suicide_prevention_compendium_5_11_20_updated-july2020.pdf**.

Additional Screening Challenges to Consider

Historically, Joint Commission field surveyors have identified compliance issues with screening for nutritional status and conducting additional assessments for individuals with eating disorders. Among surveys conducted in 2020 in BHC settings, 41.47% of organizations were cited for noncompliance with these standards.

Some Contributing Factors

Some organizations were found to have no process in place to screen for nutritional status. In some cases, staff were not clear on their facility's policy or were not trained to identify triggers that may indicate a nutritional issue requiring further assessment. Screening triggers that may warrant additional assessment include, for example, unexplained weight loss or gain, recent loss of appetite, reported difficulty eating, or uncontrolled diabetes. Because of the importance of nutritional screening, The Joint Commission requires all BHC organizations to have a policy to screen for nutritional status—regardless of setting—to identify if additional nutritional assessment is required. This is important because of the following:

- Often individuals with behavioral health issues also suffer from poor nutrition.
- Such screening may help identify an eating disorder.
- Malnutrition can manifest psychological symptoms, such as depression or inability to concentrate.
- Malnutrition can have an adverse effect on certain medications. For example, medications metabolized in the liver can have a toxic effect in individuals who are malnourished, which may lead to an overdose in malnourished individuals.

Nutritional screening may be in the form of a questionnaire completed by the individual as part of a health screening and then verified during a conversation with staff. When screening, organizations should ensure that staff are sufficiently trained in the organization's policies and practices and that such policies and practices are followed. Staff should ask all individuals questions about the following:

- Any food allergies
- Any unexplained weight loss or gain of 10 pounds or more in the last three months
- Any decrease or increase in food intake and/or appetite
- Any dental problems, such as bleeding gums, which could indicate poor nutrition
- Eating habits or behaviors that may suggest the presence of an eating disorder, such as bingeing or inducing vomiting

Screening for Trauma

Individuals seeking behavioral health care may also have experienced trauma, the effects of which often have broad implications on behavioral health long after the traumatic event has occurred. The Joint Commission defines ***trauma*** as an experience that creates a sense of fear, helplessness, or horror that overwhelms an individual's resources for coping. The impact of a traumatic event can interfere with an individual's sense of safety, ability to self-regulate, sense of self, perception of control and self-efficacy, and interpersonal relationships. Common examples of trauma experiences include sexual or physical abuse, neglect, acts of violence, and/or simply witnessing such events. Because of the devasting and long-lasting effects of trauma on individuals, The Joint Commission requires that all BHC organizations identify individuals who may have experienced trauma during initial screening and on an ongoing basis. In addition, BHC organizations are required to educate staff about trauma, abuse, neglect, and exploitation and how to refer individuals if needed. Trauma-informed care as it relates to the child welfare setting is addressed in Chapter 3.

Because of the potentially enduring negative effects trauma may have on physical and mental health, ways to address an individual's history of trauma have drawn increasing attention in recent years. A multisite project led by the Center for Health Care Strategies draws on interviews with national experts on trauma-informed care to create a framework for organizational and clinical strategies that can be implemented to address trauma. The "Successful Strategies" box below looks at ways to integrate a trauma-informed approach into an organization's care and treatment planning.

Successful Strategies

Integrating Trauma-Informed Care into Treatment Planning

Health care policy makers and providers are recognizing that exposure to traumatic events, particularly for children, heightens an individual's risk of poor physical and behavioral health long after the traumatic event. *Key Ingredients for Successful Trauma-Informed Care Implementation*, an issue brief from the Center for Health Care Strategies, takes an in-depth, evidence-based look at how organizational and clinical practices can provide a framework for implementing trauma-informed care.

Often health care providers train clinical staff in trauma-specific care but fail to implement policies and procedures necessary to implement a trauma-informed approach throughout the organization. Experts recommend that organizational reform precede clinical practices and include the following:

- **Leading and communicating about the transformational process.** Becoming a trauma-informed organization requires ongoing support from senior leaders, as it includes, for example, designating time and resources to train staff, which can influence the financial health of an organization.
- **Engaging individuals who have experienced trauma in organizational planning or programs and resources.** Individuals who have experienced trauma can provide firsthand perspective, serving alongside staff on advisory boards and boards of trustees, for example.
- **Training both clinical and nonclinical staff.** In some settings, nonclinical staff may interact with individuals served before and more frequently than clinical staff. For example, receptionists and support staff may have encounters with all individuals served. As a result, all staff, including security staff, should be trained to create a trusting, nonthreatening environment when interacting with individuals served.

- **Creating a safe environment.** A safe environment is fundamental to engaging individuals in their care and reducing the risk for retraumatization. This involves ensuring safe physical spaces, such as well-lit parking and common areas; keeping noise levels in wait areas low; and ensuring clear access to exits. It also involves ensuring a safe social-emotional environment, such as being aware of how individuals' culture affects how they perceive trauma, safety, and privacy. It also may be helpful to provide individuals with culturally relevant experiences, including foods and traditions, for example, to help create a safe emotional environment.
- **Preventing secondary traumatic stress among staff.** Emotional duress that occurs when an individual hears about the traumatic experiences of others is common among caregivers. Organizations can prevent secondary trauma among staff by developing wellness programs and encouraging staff to take mental health days off work.

Clinical practices for working with individuals who have experienced trauma include, but are not limited to, the following:

- **Involve individuals in their treatment planning and processes.** A key aspect of a trauma-informed approach is to engage individuals in their own care so that their feedback drives the direction of the care plan. This is a requirement for all individualized plans, but in a trauma-informed approach, a successful clinical practice engagement strategy may be to use peer support workers—individuals with lived trauma experiences and specialized training—as part of the care team. In this case, traumatized individuals develop trust with a peer support worker based on similar experience and shared understanding and may be more willing to engage in their own treatment planning.
- **Screen for trauma.** Trauma screening is recognized as the most fundamental aspect of a clinical trauma-informed approach, and there are many standardized trauma-informed screening tools to choose from for children and adults. Adverse childhood experiences (ACEs) are potentially traumatic events that occur in childhood (0–17 years). ACEs include events such as the following:
    - Experiencing violence, abuse, or neglect
    - Witnessing violence in the home or community
    - Having a family member attempt or die by suicide

  In addition, aspects of children's environment that may undermine their sense of safety, stability, and bonding may include growing up in a household with substance use issues, mental health problems, and instability due to parental separation or family members being incarcerated.

  Organizations should determine whether upfront and universal screening—screening every individual for trauma as early as possible—is best or to delay trauma screening after an individual has had opportunity to build trust in the provider. Decisions related to upfront screening versus delayed screening for trauma will vary depending on the setting and the individual served. The Joint Commission requires that organizations have a process for this in their policy and that they follow it. Despite varying viewpoints, the following aspects of trauma screening should be considered:
    - Treatment setting and circumstances should guide practices. For example, an emergency removal of a child from a home may dictate that screening for trauma be done after the child is settled. The time frame for screening and rescreening should be defined by the organization with respect to risk for the individual served. Individuals with a history of being abused may need to be screened frequently for any new needs.
    - Screening should benefit the individual. For example, providers who screen for trauma must ensure that they can offer appropriate care options or referral resources. For example, when screening for

trauma, if a physical health risk such as malnutrition is identified, the provider should refer the individual for further assessment and/or medical treatment, as appropriate.

- Excessive rescreening that may retraumatize the individual or cause the individual to revisit the traumatic experience should be avoided. This may require sharing screening results across treatment settings with appropriate privacy protections to help determine the need for rescreening.
- Health care professionals tasked with trauma screening should receive ample training and be proficient in conducting sensitive and appropriate follow-up discussions with respect to the individual's cultural and ethnic characteristics (for example, language, as well as cultural concepts of traumatic events).

- **Train staff in trauma-specific approaches.** Many evidence-based trauma-specific treatment approaches for children and adults exist. For example, the Trauma-Focused Cognitive Behavioral Therapy (TF-CBT) model is targeted for youth, ages 3–21, and parents or caregivers who have experienced abuse or trauma.* Whatever approach an organization selects, staff should be trained and competent in its use.

---

* US Department of Health and Human Services, Children's Bureau. *Trauma-Focused Cognitive Behavioral Therapy: A Primer for Child Welfare Professionals*. 2018. Accessed Dec 21, 2021. **https://www.childwelfare.gov/pubs/trauma/**.

Adapted from: Center for Health Care Strategies. *Key Ingredients for Successful Trauma-Informed Care Implementation*. Menschner C, Maul A. Issue Brief. Apr 2016. Accessed Dec 21, 2021. **https://www.chcs.org/resource/key-ingredients-for-successful-trauma-informed-care-implementation/**.

Summary

The process of screening individuals to identify their needs, strengths, goals, and preferences begins the groundwork for creating effective individualized treatment plans within your BHC organization. Such processes also identify an individual's risk factors and set the stage for assessment; that is, gathering more detailed data to establish whether the individual's problem requires further intervention and what that intervention should be. Chapter 2 explores the role assessment plays in the care of the individual served and how it helps confirm the presence of a problem, determines its scope and severity, and specifies treatment options for addressing the problem.

References

1. National Association of State Mental Health Program Directors. *Morbidity and Mortality in People with Serious Mental Illness*. Parks J, et al., editors. Oct 2006. Accessed Dec 21, 2021. https://www.nasmhpd.org/content/morbidity-and-mortality-people-serious-mental-illness.
2. Czeisler, ME, et al. Mental health, substance use, and suicidal ideation during the COVID-19 pandemic—United States, June 24–30, 2020. *MMWR Morb Mortal Wkly Rep*. 2020 Aug 14;69(32):1049–1057.

Tool 1-1. Plan for Care, Treatment, or Services Development Policy Template

DOWNLOAD

Tool 1-1. Sample Plan for Care, Treatment, or Services Development Policy Template			
[Logo]	**TITLE** Plan for Care, Treatment, or Services Development Policy		**IDENTIFICATION NUMBER** [Number]
ORGANIZATION(S) [Organization name]	**LEVEL** ☐ System ☐ Organization ☐ Division ☐ Department	**CATEGORY** ☐ Clinical ☐ Management ☐ Regulatory	**POSTING DATE** [MM/DD/YYYY] **EFFECTIVE DATE** [MM/DD/YYYY]
REVIEW CYCLE ☐ 1 year ☐ 3 years **LAST REVIEW DATE:** [MM/DD/YYYY]		**REPLACES** **TITLE:** Plan for Care, Treatment, or Services Development Policy **EFFECTIVE DATE(S):** [MM/DD/YYYY]	

POLICY STATEMENT

The care, treatment, or services for each individual served is guided by an individualized plan that is based on the individual's needs, strengths, preferences, and goals.

PURPOSE

To establish a process for developing individualized plans for care, treatment, or services to support coordinated care and to provide each individual served with appropriate and effective care, treatment, or services.

SCOPE

Applies to all care, treatment, or services provided by the organization.

Applies to all areas of the organization that participate in the care, treatment, or services of individuals served.

Applies to all staff members who participate in the care, treatment, or services of individuals served.
Applies to all individuals who receive care, treatment, or services from the organization.

DEFINITIONS

Adult — An individual who has reached the age of legal majority.

Assessment — 1. The process established by the organization for obtaining clinically relevant information about each individual seeking behavioral health care, treatment, or services. The information is used to match an individual's need with the appropriate setting, service/program, and intervention. 2. For opioid treatment programs, the process of identifying the precise nature and extent of a patient's substance use disorder and other medical, mental health, and social problems as a basis for treatment planning.

Continuing care/treatment/services — Care, treatment, or services provided over time in various settings, programs, or services and spanning the illness-to-wellness continuum.

Coordination of care, treatment, or services — The process of coordinating care, treatment, or services provided by an organization, including referral to appropriate community resources and liaison with others involved in care, treatment, or services (such as an individual's physician, primary care provider, or another health care organization/agency) to meet the ongoing identified needs of the individual served, to ensure implementation of the plan of care, treatment, or services, and to avoid unnecessary duplication of services.

Page 1 of 11

Discharge planning — A formalized process in an organization through which the need for a program or services of continuing and follow-up care, treatment, or services is ascertained and, if warranted, initiated for each individual served.

Family support services — A service in which family members are assigned roles and responsibilities (for example, job coach) on the support team for the patient, resident, or individual served. This term is not synonymous with family therapy/counseling.

Health information — Any information, oral or recorded, in any form or medium, that is created by a health care provider, health plan, public health authority, employer, life insurer, school or university, or health care clearinghouse that relates to past, present, or future physical or mental health or condition; the provision of health care; or payment for the provision of health care to an individual.

Health literacy — The degree to which individuals have the capacity to obtain, process, and understand basic health information and services needed to make appropriate health decisions.

Health risk behaviors — Activities undertaken by individuals that have a negative impact on their health and increase the risk of disease or injury. Examples of health risk behaviors include substance abuse, tobacco use, inadequate exercise, poor dietary practices, and unsafe sexual activity.

History and physical — Information gathered about an individual using a holistic approach for the purpose of establishing a diagnosis and developing a plan for care, treatment, or services to address physical health issues. The history may include information about previous illnesses; previous medical or surgical interventions and response to treatment; family health history; and social, cultural, economic, and lifestyle issues that may affect the individual's health and well-being. The physical involves the physical examination of the individual's body by the following means: inspection, palpation, percussion, and auscultation. When used in concert with behavioral health care services, the history and physical may be used to rule out physical causes for behavioral health conditions or to assess the impact of a medical diagnosis or treatment on a behavioral health condition.

Interpreting services — A trans-language rendition of a spoken message in which the interpreter comprehends the source language and can speak comprehensively in the target language to convey the meaning intended in the source language. The interpreter knows health and health-related terminology and provides accurate interpretations by choosing equivalent expressions that convey the best matching and meaning to the source language and captures, to the greatest possible extent, all nuances intended in the source message.

Medical history — A record consisting of an account of an individual's physical health history, obtained whenever possible from the individual, and including at least the following information: chief complaint, details of the present illness or care needs, relevant past history, and relevant inventory by body systems.

Medication reconciliation — The process of identifying the medications currently being taken by an individual. These medications are compared to newly ordered medications, and discrepancies are identified and resolved.

Minor — An individual who has not reached the age of legal majority.

Plan of care, treatment, or services — A written plan, based on data gathered during screening or assessment, that identifies care, treatment, or service needs, strengths, preferences, and goals; describes the strategy for meeting those needs, preferences, and goals; builds on the strengths and considers the preferences of the individuals served; and documents progress toward meeting the plan's objectives. The plan may include care, treatment, habilitation, and rehabilitation.

Psychosocial — Pertaining to the influence of social factors on an individual's mind or behavior and to the interrelation of behavioral and social factors.

Reassessment — Ongoing data collection, which begins on initial assessment, comparing the most recent data with the data collected at earlier assessments.

Screening — Process of determining whether individuals have certain risk factors associated with physical or behavioral health issues requiring assessment.

Translation services — A trans-language rendition of a written document in which the translator comprehends the source language and can write comprehensively in the target language to convey the meaning intended in the source language. The translator knows health and health-related terminology and provides accurate translations by choosing equivalent expressions that convey the best matching and meaning to the source language and captures, to the greatest possible extent, all nuances intended in the source document.

RESPONSIBILITIES

The Care, Treatment, and Services (CTS) Committee is responsible for the following:

- Overseeing, reviewing, revising, maintaining, and implementing this policy
- Collecting and analyzing data on compliance with this policy in collaboration with the Performance Improvement Committee

Qualified staff are responsible for performing assessments and reassessments.

Creating and maintaining an individual's plan for care, treatment, or services is the responsibility of all staff members who participate in that individual's care, treatment, or services.

PROCEDURES

Qualified staff do the following:

1. Engage the individual served in all planning activities whenever possible, including the following:
    - Screenings
    - Assessments
    - Reassessments
    - Treatment plan development
    - Discharge planning
    - Plan adjustments
    - Reevaluation of treatment plan
2. Engage the family of the individual served in plan development, unless such participation is contraindicated.
    - For adult individuals served, obtain consent from the individual served to involve family members.
    - For minor individuals served, follow applicable laws and regulations.

<u>Treatment Plan Development</u>

Staff members who participate in care, treatment, or services do the following:

1. Review and confirm information from initial screenings and assessments with the individual served and family members, if applicable.
2. Collaborate with other providers when more than one discipline is involved.
3. Collaborate with the individual served to develop a treatment plan based on the following:
    - Reason for visit
    - Clinical status (medical condition, medical problems)
    - Identified needs, strengths, preferences, and goals
    - Evidence-based practice
    - Diagnostic testing and imaging results
4. Collaborate with the individual served to identify the following:
    - Goals that capture the individual's own words or ideas
    - Goals that build on the individual's strengths

- Factors that support the transition to community integration when identified as a need during assessment
- The criteria and process for the individual's expected successful transfer and/or discharge, which the organization discusses with the individual

5. Identify the following elements related to each prioritized goal:
   - Objectives for the goal that do the following:
     - Include identified steps to achieve the goal
     - Are specific to assess the individual's progress
     - Are expressed in terms that provide the indices of progress
   - Interventions, settings, and services needed to meet the goal, including the frequency of services
   - Time frames for meeting the goal
   - Measurable metrics that will be used to determine progress
   - Potential barriers to meeting the goal and possible strategies to overcome those barriers, including consideration of the individual's strengths
   - Resources available to support the individual served in meeting the goal (for example, family support services, community agencies, financial assistance)
   - Criteria for deciding the individual served has done the following:
     - Achieved objectives for the goal
     - Met the goal
   - Discharge planning, including criteria for discharge and plans for continuing care
6. Develop next steps with the individual served.
7. Provide relevant educational materials to individuals served in a manner that meets their communication needs.
8. Confirm that the individual served understands the plan of care, treatment, or services and related information and education.
9. Document all planning activities in the individual's clinical/case record, using the individual's own words whenever possible.

Treatment Plan Review

1. Collaborate with the individual served to determine whether any components of the plan need adjusting or reevaluation, based on the following:
   - Progress of the individual served toward meeting objectives and/or prioritized goals
   - Diagnostic testing and imaging results
   - Changes to the needs, strengths, preferences, and goals of the individual served, using the individual's own words whenever possible
   - Continued relevance of the plan to the needs and goals of the individual served
2. Identify the status of the individual served with regard to the prioritized goal(s) described in the plan, including documented objectives for each goal, based on the measurable metrics described in the plan.
3. Revise the plan to reflect changes to the status of individuals and/or their needs, strengths, preferences, and/or goals.
4. Document all changes to the plan in the clinical/case record of the individual served, using the individual's own words whenever possible.

ADDITIONAL PROCEDURES FOR OPIOID TREATMENT PROGRAMS

Qualified staff do the following:

1. Follow established principles to plan for management of an individual's concurrent abuse of other drugs, when applicable.
2. Identify individuals with two or more unsuccessful withdrawal episodes within a 12-month period.
   - The program physician assesses all identified individuals to determine other potential forms of treatment.

3. Identify patients who use tobacco.
    - Include smoking and tobacco cessation as an integral part of the plan for identified individuals.
4. Identify individuals diagnosed with diseases that must be reported to public health authorities, including, but not limited to, tuberculosis and sexually transmitted diseases.
    - If appropriate to the organization's scope, include treatment for such diseases in the identified individual's plan of care, treatment, or services.
    - If treatment is outside the scope of the organization, refer the individual to another organization for further evaluation and treatment.
5. Identify the immunization status of the individual served.
    - Include free or low-cost access to immunizations recommended by the US Centers for Disease Control and Prevention, as appropriate to the individual's immunization status.
    - Provide recommended immunizations on-site, if within the organization's scope.
        - If providing recommended immunizations on-site is outside the organization's scope, provide the individual with a referral to another organization to access recommended immunizations.
6. Identify individuals diagnosed with HIV/AIDS.
    - Provide identified individuals with information about community HIV/AIDS treatment programs, prevention programs, and social support services.

ADDITIONAL PROCEDURES FOR ORGANIZATIONS PROVIDING CARE, TREATMENT, OR SERVICES TO CHILDREN OR YOUTH

Qualified staff do the following:

1. Assess the educational needs of each child or youth served.
2. Identify individuals whose care, treatment, or services will cause a significant absence from school.
3. Include educational services in the plan for identified individuals, in accordance with laws and regulations.

ADDITIONAL PROCEDURES FOR ORGANIZATIONS PROVIDING EMPLOYMENT ASSISTANCE

Qualified staff do the following:

1. Address the following elements in the individual's plan of care, treatment, or services:
    - Preparing the individual for employment
    - Gaining employment
    - Maintaining employment
    - Improving employment

ADDITIONAL PROCEDURES FOR ORGANIZATIONS PROVIDING VOCATIONAL REHABILITATION SERVICES

Qualified staff do the following:

1. Include in the individual's plan of care, treatment, or services the needs, skills, preferences, and goals related to the following:
    - Job training
    - Securing employment

ADDITIONAL PROCEDURES FOR ORGANIZATIONS THAT USE ACTIVITY THERAPIES

Qualified staff do the following:

1. Include in the individual's plan of care, treatment, or services any activity therapies used to support achievement of a specific goal(s).

ADDITIONAL PROCEDURES FOR ORGANIZATIONS THAT USE ANIMAL-ASSISTED THERAPY

Qualified staff do the following:

1. Assess all individuals to determine the following:

    - Whether they are candidates for animal-assisted therapy
    - Whether they have contraindications to animal-assisted therapy
2. Include relevant information in the individual's plan of care, treatment, or services.

ADDITIONAL PROCEDURES FOR ORGANIZATIONS PROVIDING FAMILY SUPPORT SERVICES

Qualified staff do the following:

1. Assess the role of family members and their access to information.
    - Base this assessment on the age of the individual served and applicable laws and regulations.
2. Engage family members providing support in developing the plan for care, treatment, or services, when indicated by the individual served.
3. Identify the roles and participation of family members providing support in the plan for care, treatment, or services.

ADDITIONAL PROCEDURES FOR ORGANIZATIONS PROVIDING PEER SUPPORT

Qualified staff do the following:

1. Identify the amount of information that can be accessed by peers providing support, as determined by the individual served.
2. Identify the involvement of peers providing support, as determined by the individual served.
3. Include the above information in the individual's plan of care, treatment, or services.

ADDITIONAL PROCEDURES FOR ORGANIZATIONS PROVIDING CASE MANAGEMENT/CARE COORDINATION SERVICES

Qualified staff do the following:

1. Engage the individual served in service planning.
2. Engage the family members of the individual served in service planning, if appropriate.
3. Identify the needs, preferences, and goals of the individual served as related to the following elements:
    - Housing
    - Employment
    - Education
    - Transportation
    - Crisis support
    - Health care and behavioral health services
    - Financial services and benefits
    - Assistance with housekeeping
    - Assistance with personal hygiene
    - Assistance with retention and improvement of skills related to daily living
    - Social support and adaptive skills
    - Support of spirituality
    - Schools
    - Leisure and recreational activities for all individuals
    - Parental support for children and youth
    - Interaction with the criminal or juvenile justice system, if applicable
4. Identify family, neighborhood, and community support and services to assist individuals served in meeting their goals.
5. Document the above information in the individual's plan of care, treatment, or services.

ADDITIONAL PROCEDURES FOR ORGANIZATIONS PROVIDING COMMUNITY INTEGRATION SERVICES

Qualified staff do the following:

1. Identify the following, in accordance with the needs, preferences, and goals of the individual served:
    - Type of education, training, and support provided

- Intensity of education, training, and support provided
- Duration of education, training, and support provided

2. Identify educational opportunities to be provided to individuals, in accordance with their needs, preferences, and goals. These opportunities include the following:
    - Personal grooming and hygiene
    - Housekeeping
    - Shopping for necessities
    - Meal preparation and healthy eating
    - Budgeting
    - Banking
    - Accessing public transportation
    - Use of community resources
    - Communication skills
    - Social skills
    - Leisure and recreational activities for children, youth, and adults
    - Volunteer activity
    - Illness self-management (for example, symptom management, medication management), including what to do in case of a health crisis or urgent health problem
3. Document the above information in the individual's plan of care, treatment, or services.

Additional Procedures for Organizations That Elect The Joint Commission Behavioral Health Home Option

The integrated care team does the following:

1. Engages the individual served in service planning.
2. Engages the family members of the individual served in service planning, if appropriate.
3. Identifies the needs, preferences, and goals of the individual served as related to the following elements:
    - Housing
    - Employment
    - Education
    - Transportation
    - Crisis support
    - Integrated health services
    - Illness self-management (for example, symptom management, medication management), including what to do in case of a health crisis or urgent health problem
    - Habilitation and rehabilitation services
    - Financial services and benefits
    - Assistance with housekeeping
    - Assistance with personal hygiene
    - Assistance with the retention and improvement of other skills related to activities of daily living
    - Social support and adaptive skills
    - Support of spirituality
    - Schools
    - Leisure and recreational activities
    - Parental support for children and youth
    - Interaction with the criminal or juvenile justice system, if applicable
4. Identifies family, neighborhood, and community supports and services to assist individuals served in meeting their goals.
5. Documents the above information in the individual's plan of care, treatment, or services.

REFERENCES

Joint Commission Standard CTS.02.01.03. The organization performs screenings and assessments as defined by the organization's policy.

Joint Commission Standard CTS.02.01.05. **For organizations providing care, treatment, or services in non-24-hour settings:** The organization implements a written process requiring a physical health screening to determine the individual's need for a medical history and physical examination.

Joint Commission Standard CTS.02.01.07, Element of Performance (EP) 5. **For opioid treatment programs:** The program documents the patient's medical and family history to determine current chronic or acute medical conditions, such as diabetes; renal diseases; hepatitis A, B, C, and D; HIV exposure; tuberculosis; sexually transmitted diseases; other infectious diseases; sickle-cell trait or anemia; pregnancy (including past history of pregnancy and current involvement in prenatal care); and chronic cardiopulmonary disease.

Joint Commission Standard CTS.02.01.07, EP 6. **For opioid treatment programs:** Based on the patient's history and physical examination, the program evaluates the possibility of various conditions (such as infectious disease, liver or pulmonary conditions, cardiac abnormalities, psychiatric problems, dermatologic sequelae of addiction, and concurrent surgical problems).

Joint Commission Standard CTS.02.01.07, EP 8. **For opioid treatment programs:** The program immunizes the patient, or refers the patient for immunization, against hepatitis A and B if not already immune, and against other viral hepatitis strains as those vaccines become available.

Joint Commission Standard CTS.02.01.09. The organization screens all individuals served for physical pain.

Joint Commission Standard CTS.02.01.11. The organization screens all individuals served for their nutritional status.

Joint Commission Standard CTS.02.02.01, EP 6. Family members are invited to participate in the assessment process as relevant to the care, treatment, or services provided, and the age and preference of the individual served.

Joint Commission Standard CTS.02.02.07. The organization reassesses individuals served, as needed.

Joint Commission Standard CTS.02.03.01. **For organizations providing care, treatment, or services to a child or youth:** The organization facilitates and coordinates family or guardian involvement throughout the assessment process.

Joint Commission Standard CTS.03.01.01, EP 1. In collaboration with the individual served and, as appropriate, their family, the organization makes care, treatment, or service decisions that are based on information it has collected about the individual's needs, strengths, preferences, and goals.

Joint Commission Standard CTS.03.01.03. The organization has a plan for care, treatment, or services that reflects the assessed needs, strengths, preferences, and goals of the individual served.

Joint Commission Standard CTS.03.01.05, EP 1. The family of the individual served is involved in developing the plan for care, treatment, or services upon consent from the individual (if an adult) or in accordance with law and regulation (if a minor), unless such participation is contraindicated. Family participation is documented.

Page 8 of 11

Joint Commission Standard CTS.04.02.13, EP 1. **For organizations providing care, treatment, or services to children or youth:** The organization defines the length of stay and absence from school that would require providing educational services in accordance with applicable law and regulation.

Joint Commission Standard CTS.04.03.01, EP 1. **For organizations providing employment assistance:** The organization assists the individual served in the following:

- Determining the individual's desire to work
- Identifying the individual's personal interests, values, and vocational preferences
- Identifying the individual's employment needs
- Identifying or refining the individual's employment goal
- Identifying employment opportunities (for example, reviewing employment ads, browsing the Internet), and in preparations to secure employment (for example, preparing résumé, completing applications)
- Developing the skills and supports needed to maintain employment

Joint Commission Standard CTS.04.03.05, EP 5. **For organizations that provide vocational rehabilitation services:** The organization assists the individual served in assessing the following related to securing and maintaining employment:

- The individual's expectations for the personal, financial, and social benefits of working
- The individual's aptitudes, interests, and motivations toward involvement in various job-related activities
- The individual's desire for career planning assistance

Joint Commission Standard CTS.04.03.13, EP 1. **For organizations that provide vocational rehabilitation services:** The organization assists the individual served in developing a plan for employment that focuses on the individual's employment goals and objectives.

Joint Commission Standard CTS.04.03.13, EP 2. **For organizations that provide vocational rehabilitation services:** The organization develops a written employment plan that is specific to the individual served.

Joint Commission Standard CTS.04.03.17. **For organizations that use activity therapies:** Activity therapies that are used to support achievement of a specific goal(s) are incorporated into the plan for care, treatment, or services.

Joint Commission Standard CTS.04.03.21, EP 1. **For organizations that use animal-assisted therapy:** Each individual is assessed to determine whether they are a candidate for animal- assisted therapy and whether the individual has any contraindications to animal-assisted therapy.

Joint Commission Standard CTS.04.03.27. **For organizations providing family support services:** The plan for care, treatment, or services identifies the role of families.

Joint Commission Standard CTS.04.03.31. **For organizations providing peer support:** The plan for care, treatment, or services addresses the involvement of peer support when provided.

Joint Commission Standard CTS.06.01.01, EP 1. **For organizations providing case management/care coordination services:** The individual served and, as appropriate, their family, are partners with organization staff in service planning.

Joint Commission Standard CTS.06.01.01, EP 2. **For organizations providing case management/care coordination services:** With the assistance of staff, the individual served and, as appropriate, their family, identify needs, preferences, and goals for the following:

- Housing

- Employment
- Education
- Transportation
- Crisis support
- Health care and behavioral health services (for example, medication, therapy)
- Financial services and benefits
- Assistance with housekeeping
- Assistance with personal hygiene
- Assistance with the retention and improvement of other skills related to activities of daily living
- Social support and adaptive skills
- Support of spirituality
- Schools
- Leisure and recreational activities for children, youth, and adults
- Parental support for children and youth
- Interaction with the criminal or juvenile justice system, if applicable

Joint Commission Standard CTS.06.01.01, EP 3. **For organizations providing case management/care coordination services:** Staff coordinating case management/care coordination services assist the individual served in identifying, using, and accessing family, neighborhood, and community supports and services.

Joint Commission Standard CTS.06.01.03. **For organizations providing community integration services:** The individual served, with assistance from the organization, determines their needs and wants for education, training, and support to help their progress toward independent living and community integration.

Joint Commission Standard CTS.06.01.07. **For organizations that elect The Joint Commission Behavioral Health Home option:** The individual served, with assistance from the organization, determines their needs, preferences, and goals regarding training and support to help them progress toward independent living and community integration.

Joint Commission Standard RC.02.01.01, EP 4. As needed to provide care, treatment, or services, the clinical/case record contains the following additional information:

- Any advance directives
- Any informed consent
- Any documentation of protective services
- Any documentation of consent by the individual served, family, or guardian for admission; care, treatment, or services; evaluation; continuing care; or research
- Any records of communication with the individual served, such as telephone calls or e-mail
- Any documentation of involvement in care, treatment, or services by the individual served and, when necessary, their family
- Any information on unusual occurrences, such as complications; accidents or injuries to the individual served; procedures that place the individual served at risk or cause pain; other illnesses or conditions that affect care, treatment, or services; or the death of the individual served
- Any indications for and episodes of special procedures

Joint Commission Standard RI.01.02.01, EP 1. The organization involves the individual served in making decisions about their care, treatment, or services.

Joint Commission Standard RI.01.02.01, EP 8. The individual served has the right to involve their family in decisions about care, treatment, or services. When there is a surrogate decision-maker, the surrogate can exercise the right to involve the family on behalf of the individual served, in accordance with law and regulation.

Companion Policies
Discharge Planning Policy
Medication Reconciliation Policy
Screening, Assessment, and Reassessment Policy

APPROVAL

NAME AND CREDENTIALS [Name and Credentials] **TITLE** [Title]	**NAME AND CREDENTIALS** [Name and Credentials] **TITLE** [Title]	
SIGNATURE		**DATE** [MM/DD/YYYY]
SIGNATURE		**DATE** [MM/DD/YYYY]

Chapter 2
The Role of Assessment in the Individualized Plan

Relevant Standards Covered in This Chapter	
CTS.03.01.03	The organization has a plan for care, treatment, or services that reflects the assessed needs, strengths, preferences, and goals of the individual served.
	EP 1 The organization develops a plan for care, treatment, or services that reflects the assessed needs, strengths, preferences, and goals of the individual served.
	EP 2 The plan for care, treatment, or services includes the following: • Goals that are expressed in a manner that captures the individual's words or ideas • Goals that build on the individual's strengths • Factors that support the transition to community integration when identified as a need during assessment • The criteria and process for the individual's expected successful transfer and/or discharge/termination of services, which the organization discusses with the individual (For more information, refer to Standard CTS.06.02.01) **Note 1:** Barriers that might need to be considered include co-occurring illnesses, cognitive and communicative disorders, developmental disabilities, vision or hearing disabilities, physical disabilities, and social and environmental factors.
	EP 3 The objectives of the plan for care, treatment, or services meet the following criteria: • They are based on identified goals • They include identified steps to achieve the goal(s) • They are sufficiently specific to assess the progress of the individual served • They are expressed in terms that provide indices of progress
	EP 4 The organization reevaluates and, when necessary, revises the goals and objectives of the plan for care, treatment, or services based on change(s) in the individual's needs, preferences, and goals and the individual's response to care, treatment, or services. If no change(s) occurs, the goals and objectives are reevaluated at a specified time interval established by organization policy.
	EP 5 Reasons for deferring a goal, or the objectives leading toward or related to a goal, are documented.
	EP 6 The organization provides care, treatment, or services for each individual served according to the plan for care, treatment, or services.

Relevant Standards Covered in This Chapter	
CTS.03.01.05	The plan for care, treatment, or services addresses the family's involvement.
	EP 1 The family of the individual served is involved in developing the plan for care, treatment, or services upon consent from the individual (if an adult) or in accordance with law and regulation (if a minor), unless such participation is contraindicated. Family participation is documented. (*See also* CTS.04.02.16, EP 5)
CTS.03.01.07	When individuals served need additional care, treatment, or services not offered by the organization, referrals are made and documented in the clinical/case record. (For more information, refer to Standard CTS.04.01.01.)

Note: Joint Commission standards are updated on a regular basis. Always refer to the most current version of the *Comprehensive Accreditation Manual for Behavioral Health Care and Human Services* (*CAMBHC*) or its E-dition® counterpart for requirements relevant to your setting.

Terms to Know

assessment
diagnostic summary, or summary statement
goals
interdisciplinary
interventions
motivational interviewing
objectives
Patient Health Questionnaire-9 (PHQ-9)
Generalized Anxiety Disorder-7 (GAD-7) Questionnaire
reassessment
shared decision making

Introduction

In Chapter 1 we discussed the importance of effective screening to help lay the foundation for individualized treatment planning. We explored various screening tools and addressed some challenges behavioral health care and human services (BHC) organizations often have with Joint Commission screening standards. In this chapter we explore assessment and reassessment as a way to evaluate the individual served in more depth and confirm the presence of a problem, its scope and severity, and treatment options for addressing the problem. We take a look at using assessment data in treatment planning to develop the individual's goals and objectives. We also look at the importance of reassessing individuals when reviewing the treatment plan to help monitor an individual's progress in care.

As discussed in Chapter 1, **assessment** is the process of collecting, analyzing, and prioritizing all information relevant to developing an effective and individualized treatment plan for an individual seeking behavioral health care or services. The purpose of assessment is to match the individual's needs with the appropriate setting, service, program, and intervention for a positive outcome. Assessment practices should help further identify an individual's strengths and preferences to help practitioners select the best resources for addressing an individual's problems. Assessment data will vary as the organization determines—based on its service and setting—the content and format of an individual's assessment and how frequently that individual should be reassessed. For example, a substance use assessment will evaluate the severity and nature of a substance use disorder and may also explore the possibility of co-occurring disorders. During the assessment, other factors should be evaluated including the individual's friends, family, or support network, marital, interpersonal, physical, and spiritual life; financial and legal situations; and any other issues that might affect treatment and recovery. In addition, because individuals are complex and rarely have only one problem, assessment helps identify if someone with a substance use issue also has depression, or if someone with an eating disorder might also have experienced trauma, for example. A goal of assessment is to get a complete picture of the individual served by considering all needs, goals, strengths, and preferences and then prioritizing data to inform appropriate care.

Assessment involves not just analyzing data collected during screening but also obtaining clinically relevant information, such as the *severity* of an individual's disorder, for example, which may be determined by using various instruments and tools. Several evidence-based assessment tools will be discussed later in this chapter, which are designed to drive treatment decisions. BHC organizations must determine the content and format of the assessment based on their services and settings. Depending on the population served, The Joint Commission has specific assessment requirements for particular populations served, including the following:

- Care, Treatment, and Services (CTS) Standard CTS.02.02.01, Elements of Performance (EPs) 7–9, for organizations certified as Behavioral Health Homes (includes short and long-term health goals; chronic physical health conditions, such as diabetes, hypertension, and heart disease, to name a few; and the individual's ability to self-manage identified chronic conditions)
- CTS.02.02.07, EP 2, and CTS.02.02.09 for opioid treatment programs (assessments are updated quarterly during individual's first year of continuous treatment and semiannually subsequently and include toxicology tests and medical assessment to monitor and evaluate an individual's treatment progress)
- CTS.02.03.03 for Children and Youth (includes legal custody status, the child's development as related to chronological age, the child's recreational interests, family history and dynamics as related to the child's current needs and discharge planning)
- CTS.02.03.05 for Individuals with intellectual/ development disabilities (includes cognitive and physical functioning needs, family support, independent living skills and interests, and intelligence testing, to name a few)
- CTS.02.03.09 and CTS.02.03.11 for eating disorders treatment (includes the individual's beliefs, perceptions, attitudes, and behavior regarding food as well as any laboratory tests, as determined by the organization and in accordance with the level of care provided)
- CTS.02.03.07 and CTS.02.03.13 for addictions treatment (includes the individual's history of addiction, readiness to change, current living arrangement and environment, as well as options for an alternative and supportive environment, as needed)

Always check the most current version of the *CAMBHC* or E-dition® for assessment requirements applicable to services provided.

Prioritizing Needs for Assessment

To maintain a person-centered focus, clinicians and qualified BHC professionals should actively engage the individual served when analyzing and prioritizing needs identified during screening. The assessment process allows the individual to validate information shared during screening as accurate and complete, but it also can be used to address and prioritize immediate needs for care, treatment, or services. For example, if—during a thorough assessment of an individual seeking help for an eating disorder—the individual shows signs of malnutrition, such as feeling tired or cold most of the time, having wounds that take a long time to heal, and/or poor concentration, that individual may require immediate referral to a medical health provider for physical medical treatment.

All data from screening and assessment should be gathered, analyzed, and interpreted. It is good practice to then consolidate such data into a **diagnostic summary, or summary statement**. Although, often called a diagnostic summary, it may go by a variety of other names, such as clinical or case formulation or impression, conclusions, or recommendations. A multidisciplinary team or a single practitioner may create the diagnostic summary. It should reflect and document the clinicians' analyses of data and identify and prioritize expressed needs to further develop the treatment plan. Such a summary may be included in the plan for care and updated as needed.

Figure 2-1 illustrates how screening and assessment data for an individual—which take into account the individual's needs, strengths, and preferences—identify and prioritize needs to help formulate a diagnostic summary. The purpose of creating a diagnostic summary is not to reiterate data points but to drive progress forward in developing the individualized treatment plan. A diagnostic summary should include the following:

- Assessed needs, strengths, preferences, and goals (for example, the individual admitted for anger management, likes to draw, has a good work ethic, and prefers to work on his own rather than in a group)

- Relevant historical data and background information (for example, the individual is obese and has type 2 diabetes but also has family and community health services support to assist with recovery)
- Interpretation of information gathered (intervention will primarily focus on the individual's anger in response to bullying and his comfort level with being in groups; however, the need to express himself through drawing may be revisited as an intervention to help manage anger)

It is important for behavioral health care professionals to remember that assessment processes help identify what screening data are most meaningful to the care, treatment, or service of the individual served. Also, when clinicians involve the individual in the assessment process, it inspires dialogue that provides additional insight into the individual's needs, strengths, preferences, and goals and continues to lay groundwork for an effective treatment plan. Remember that collaboration also improves engagement with the individual and inspires ownership of the treatment plan, which leads to better adherence to the plan and better overall outcomes.

Importance of Reassessment

The importance of reassessing individuals as part of treatment planning cannot be overstated. Reassessing individuals served throughout the course of care, treatment, and services is critical to monitoring progress toward identified goals. Under Standard CTS.03.01.09, which is related to measurement-based care and is discussed in more detail in Chapter 3, The Joint Commission requires all BHC organizations to assess outcomes of care, treatment, or services provided to the individual served. The best way to do this is to monitor the individuals' progress by reassessing them throughout the course of care. Organizations are required to define their reassessment practices in their policies, the scope of which will vary depending on the individual's functioning, the organization's setting and scope of service, the individual's preferences, and the individual's response to treatment. The purposes of **reassessment** include the following:

- To evaluate the individual's response to care, treatment, or services
- To address changes in the individual's status and/or diagnosis or condition

Figure 2-1. Prioritizing Needs to Form a Diagnostic Summary

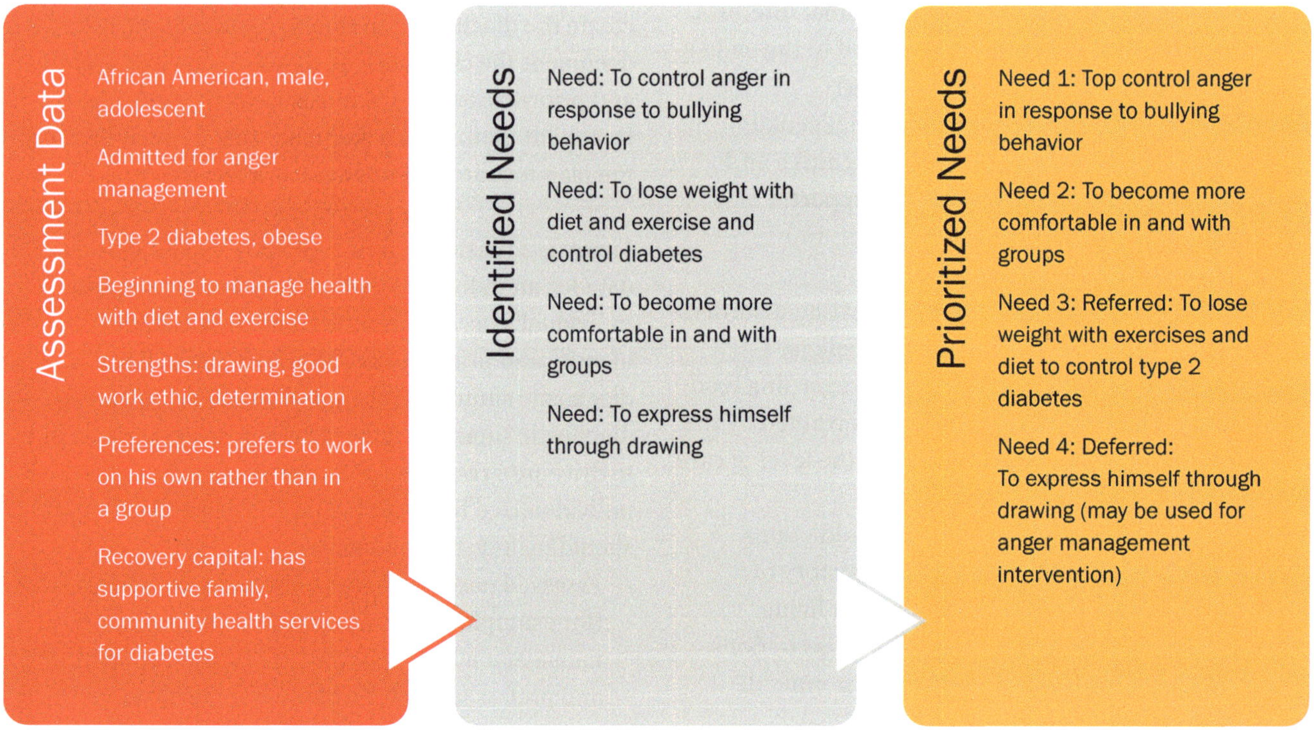

- To satisfy legal or regulatory requirements
- To meet designated time intervals for treatment plan review, as determined by organization policies
- To meet designated intervals as determined by the individual's course of care, treatment, or services

Using Assessment and Reassessment Tools

To capture and prioritize information related to individuals' needs, strengths, preferences, and goals throughout their care, treatment, and services, organizations may choose to use a variety of assessment tools, including questionnaires, forms, psychological tests, and so on, to help plan individualized treatment and interventions. Organizations are required to choose tools appropriate for the population served. For example, if an organization provides treatment for depression, its assessment tools should be designed for that diagnosis. The Joint Commission does not prescribe the use of any particular tool. However, for compliance with Joint Commission requirements related to measurement-based care, such tools should be standardized to monitor an individual's progress, validated, reliable, and evidence-based, as discussed in Chapter 3.

For example, many BHC organizations use the **Patient Health Questionnaire-9 (PHQ-9)** as a tool to assess and monitor levels of depression in an individual. The questionnaire contains nine questions. Each response is assigned a score, which determines the individual's depression severity, as shown in the table below:

PHQ-9 Score	Depression Severity
0–4	None–minimal
5–9	Mild
10–14	Moderate
15–19	Moderately severe
20–27	Severe

Individuals' PHQ-9 score helps determine their treatment and intervention option, which is based on the most effective level of care required for the severity of depression. The PHQ-9 can be administered as part of an organization's initial screening and assessment processes, throughout the course of treatment to reassess and monitor change, and at discharge to evaluate outcomes of care. The PHQ-9 is just one frequently used assessment tool to address one diagnostic category (depression) that can also be used for reassessment and monitoring an individual's progress (a sample PHQ-9 is provided in Tool 2-1 on page 48).

Another commonly used assessment and monitoring tool is the **Generalized Anxiety Disorder-7 (GAD-7) Questionnaire**, which consists of seven items, responses to which are assigned a score to evaluate severity levels for generalized anxiety. A sample GAD-7 is provided on page 49. An individuals' level of anxiety or severity is determined by their total score as shown in the table below.

GAD-7 Score	Anxiety Severity
0–5	Mild
6–10	Moderate
11–15	Moderately severe
15–21	Severe anxiety

Chapter 3 includes an example of how the PHQ-9 can be used to meet Joint Commission requirements for outcomes-based care. In addition, practical use of the PHQ-9 is included in the sample treatment plan in Chapter 5.

Evaluating Assessment Strategies

To reduce deficiencies in assessment processes, it may be useful to design checklists that capture your organization's assessment policy requirements as well as the data requirements set forth by state law, regulatory agencies, insurance providers, accreditors, and other stakeholders. Although many BHC organizations use an electronic health record (EHR) and may have limited ability to influence its design, it is a good practice, to any extent possible, to include prompts within EHR assessment documentation to ensure that all required elements are addressed. Review the sample questions listed in the "Successful Strategies" box on page 40 as a starting point for evaluating your organization's assessment forms and practices. These questions may provide guidance for improving assessment forms, creating checklists, and including prompts to support your facility's assessment processes.

Successful Strategies

Evaluating Your Assessment Forms

When evaluating your organization's assessment forms, ask yourself the following:

- ☐ Does this form capture all the information required, in appropriate detail, for an accurate screening or assessment for the types of individuals served by my BHC organization?
- ☐ Does it comply with all applicable regulatory requirements for screening/assessments, including state and federal laws?
- ☐ Does it comply with all applicable stakeholder requirements (such as insurance carriers, grant providers, and so on) for screening/assessments?
- ☐ Does it comply with Joint Commission requirements for your setting/services?
- ☐ Do the sections and questions follow a logical progression?
- ☐ Do the questions promote concise, clear responses?
- ☐ Is there enough room to document direct quotes from the individual served, family members, and other sources of information? (Remember that The Joint Commission requires that treatment plans use the words/language of the individual served to capture goals, needs, strengths, and preferences.)
- ☐ Is there a system for distinguishing between facts or hard data, observations, and opinions? For example, is there an option to indicate the source of any information (self-reported, reported by family, reported in medical record, observed by BHC professional, and so on) for any particular question and a place to document such a source?
- ☐ Do the data collected support the diagnosis, condition, or description of symptoms and current functioning of the individual?
- ☐ Are there any missing data? Remember that evaluating your assessments form means looking at what it includes and what may be missing.
- ☐ After reading the assessment, do you know how the individual served would like life to improve? Is that goal expressed in the individual's own words/language?
- ☐ If the individual served has received previous care, treatment, or services, can you tell from reading the assessment what the individual's preferences are and what has worked in the past?
- ☐ After reading the assessment, can you describe what factors need to be addressed (such as skills learned, fears reduced, and resources developed) to facilitate improvement?

When evaluating your organization's practices related to assessment forms:

- ☐ Do all clinicians and staff across your organization complete the form correctly and consistently?
- ☐ Are all clinicians and staff trained in how to use assessment forms upon orientation?
- ☐ If a clinician or staff member is not properly or consistently using assessments forms, how is that identified?
- ☐ Are forms easily accessible by clinicians and staff when needed?
- ☐ Are clinicians and staff encouraged to offer their feedback on use of forms, whether they are satisfied with them, and ways to improve the forms, if needed?
- ☐ Does your organization have a process for reviewing the effectiveness and completion of assessment forms?

Including Identified Goals and Measurable Objectives

Treatment plans should be driven by the individual's identified **goals** for a positive outcome and include measurable objectives for achieving those goals. However, it is important to ensure that the individual's goals are realistic. This may require some refinement during collaborative discussions between the individual and the clinician. For example, an individual's goal may be to live independently, even though that individual is unemployed and has no source of income. As a result, the goal, as stated, is not immediately achievable. It may, however, be identified as a long-term goal or a deferred goal, with measurable objectives based on the individual's current level of care.

A goal is the end point of care, treatment, or services in relation to an identified need. It is reached when the individual achieves optimal and acceptable resolution of the need.

Some common behavioral health goals may include the following:

- I need to stop drinking alcohol daily.
- I want to improve my relationship with my son.
- I want to feel less anxious.
- I need to improve my physical health.

Several examples of individual goals are included in the sample treatment plans in Chapter 5. When collaborating with an individual served to develop treatment plan goals, keep in mind that Joint Commission–compliant treatment plans must include goals that meet the following criteria:

- They capture the individual's words and ideas.
- They build on the individual's strengths.
- They include factors that support transition to community integration when identified as a need during assessment.
- They include criteria and processes for the individual's expected successful transfer and/or discharge/termination of services.
- They address any barriers to consider, such as co-occurring illnesses, cognitive and communicative disorders, developmental disabilities, vision or hearing disabilities, physical disabilities, and social and environmental factors.
- They include identified and measurable objectives for achieving the goal.

To effectively monitor and track an individual's progress, treatment plans must include measurable and time-bound objectives for achieving identified goals. **Objectives** are actionable behaviors that help individuals reach their goals. Examples of treatment plan objectives tied to specific goals are provided in the sample treatment plans in Chapter 5. Other objectives may include actions performed outside the treatment environment, such as the following:

- For someone with a goal of improving her relationship with her son, an objective might be to count to 10 before speaking and avoid using hurtful words (curse words, name calling, and so on) during arguments or disagreements.
- For someone who has a goal to reduce their anxiety, the objective might be to turn off screens and listen to classical music before bedtime every night.
- For someone with a goal to control/stop/recover from an addiction, the objective could be to discard items that trigger addiction behaviors (for example, lighters, drug paraphernalia, candy, gambling apps, gift cards to fast food restaurants).
- For someone with a goal to improve self-esteem, the objective may be to practice three new coping skills in three weeks and use those learned skills when negative thoughts are triggered.

Objectives must relate specifically to identified goals. Compliant treatment plans should include objectives that meet the following criteria:

- They identify steps and time frames to achieve the individual's goals.
- They are sufficiently specific to assess the progress of the individual served.
- They are expressed in terms that provide indexes of progress.

Common Challenges with Goals and Objectives

Joint Commission surveyors commonly cite organizations for noncompliance for including goals and objectives in the treatment plan that are not expressed in the individual's words or ideas. To combat this, the "Successful Strategies" box on page 42 offers one approach to encouraging collaborative goal setting with individuals who may have difficulty expressing their goals (for example, children).

Joint Commission surveyors also report that many treatment plans do not contain goals and objectives, or the objectives noted have no relationship to identified goals. In addition, although it may not be necessary to capture the individual's goals verbatim, there must be evidence within the treatment plan that the words and ideas expressed by the individual served are not scripted or expressed in language that might apply to several different individuals. For example, a goal that reads "the individual wants to establish a loving relationship with her son" is an example of scripted language; whereas, a goal that reads "I want to get along better with my son and not fight all the time" may ring more true for that individual. As such, treatment plans should include language the individual could easily express and understand (based on the individual's education or cognitive level). In addition, during treatment planning, individuals may be assisted to develop measurable objectives for realizing their goal. For example, the individual may express "I will meditate every day." During discussion with the individual, such an objective can be made measurable and include indices for progress, such as "I will wake 15 minutes earlier every day to build in time to add meditation to my morning schedule."

Collaborative and Interdisciplinary Treatment Plans

In driving and identifying delivery of care, The Joint Commission requires that the organization collaborate with individuals served (and, as appropriate, their families) when making decisions that drive interventions and delivery of care. In addition, an individual's words and ideas must be incorporated into treatment plan goals and objectives. Organizations must also build on that individual's strengths and address barriers to achievement. One way to ensure collaborative treatment planning is to implement organization policies based on shared decision making.

Successful Strategies

Motivational Interviewing for Collaborative Goal Setting

It can be difficult for some, particularly preadolescents, adolescents, and those individuals remanded to treatment by health or legal authorities, to engage in a collaborative goal-setting process. One evidence-based approach designed to encourage individuals to talk themselves into making beneficial changes is **motivational interviewing**. This client-centered technique is based on principles of the humanistic psychology of Carl Rogers and helps manifest open dialogue in a psychologically safe environment. It includes encouraging individuals to think and talk about their reasons to change by doing the following:

- Asking open-ended questions. *What makes you feel stressed out?*
- Affirming dialog. *It sounds like what you described is a real challenge.*
- Using reflective listening. *What I hear you say is that you feel most stressed before school.*
- Summarizing. Encouraging youth to reflect on the core ideas of the story they describe. *I think you should think about the ways you can calm yourself and alleviate your stress while at school, considering what you shared about your teacher and classmates with me.*

Using motivational interviewing can help elicit a collaborative process of careful cultivation of individuals' beliefs in their ability to grow.

Source: Adapted from PositivePsychology.com. 17 Motivational Interviewing Questions and Skills. Souders B. Accessed Dec 22, 2021. **https://positivepsychology.com/motivational-interviewing/**.

A widely used definition of ***shared decision making*** in mental health is "a process in which clinicians and patients work together to select tests, treatments, management or support packages, based on clinical evidence and the [individual's] informed preferences. It involves the provision of evidence-based information about options, outcomes and uncertainties, together with decision support counseling and a system for recording and implementing [individuals'] informed preferences"[1(p. vii)a]

Treatment plans must also be **interdisciplinary** whenever more than one discipline is involved in the care, treatment, or services of an individual. In other words, the treatment plan is not the work of just one professional. It must involve all professional disciplines, determined both by the structure of the treatment program and the individual's identified needs, goals, and objectives. There is a hierarchical structure, in which the intervention and the discipline providing the intervention have a clearly identified role in helping to achieve the individual's objectives, which are linked to a treatment goal. The critical factor is to identify, within the treatment plan, the role of each discipline involved in the intervention that is designed to achieve the individual's objectives. Here is an example:

- Individual's goal: "I want to sleep better."
- Objectives:
  - The individual will spend a half hour before bedtime engaging in a relaxing activity to prepare for sleep, such as meditation, listening to music, or reading.
  - The individual will log quality of sleep daily in the morning.
  - **Therapist** will provide education on progressive relaxation techniques and will check in with the individual at each session on quality of sleep and review the individual record in the log.
  - **Therapist** will help the individual identify and practice 1–2 relaxing activities (for example, listening to quiet music, mindfulness exercise) and will assist the individual in developing a log to track results.
  - **Psychiatrist** will prescribe anti-anxiety medication that will function as a sleep aid and will monitor the appropriate dosage based on the quality of the sleep log kept by the individual.

Objectives will require involvement from different disciplines relative to identified steps, but all objectives should track back to the target goals for all disciplines. In other words, everyone should be working toward the same treatment goals regardless of their specific role and tasks, as opposed to operating on parallel tracks that may not relate to the individual's identified goals. For some individuals' goals, multiple disciplines may play a part, while in others, it may be some but not all disciplines, as appropriate. In the example above, if the individual has a medical condition, such as sleep apnea, which interferes with restorative sleep, a physician would need to be identified and included in the treatment plan to address the sleep apnea condition and its effect on the individual's goal to sleep better.

Reevaluating and Revising Plan Goals and Objectives

For Joint Commission compliance, goals and objectives should be reevaluated regularly—even if no change occurs—at specified intervals established by the BHC organization's policy. Please note that The Joint Commission does not specify the frequency with which goals and objectives are reevaluated; that is determined by the BHC organization itself. And Joint Commission surveyors then observe and determine if the BHC organization is following its own policy regarding frequency and timing of reevaluation and revision of plan goals and objectives. Health care organizations often don't realize that their own policies and procedures are what Joint Commission surveyors are looking at to determine the organization's compliance, depending on the situation. When a significant issue has surfaced that may identify a new need, strength, and/or preference, the clinician and the individual served must decide whether the new need is to be added to the treatment plan. For example, what if an individual has been in treatment for two months for anxiety and depression, but then the individual is laid off from work, which then triggers increasing depression and thoughts of suicide in the individual? Because the employment change created a new problem for the individual served, it would warrant a change in the treatment plan that includes the addition of new goals.

Whenever changes occur, an existing treatment plan should be revised. If the case notes, over time, suggest that no significant change has occurred, or that the individual's condition has worsened, a review of the treatment plan is warranted to determine where changes can be made in the plan. It is important for practitioners to identify reasons for an individual's progress—or lack of progress—and adjust goals and objectives accordingly.

The Joint Commission requires that the plan be reviewed for updates according to a time frame set by the organization. Even if no change occurs, the goals and objectives must be reevaluated at a specified time frame established within the organization's policy—whether the individual has improved or not. In some cases, stakeholders, including insurance companies and regulators, may require review of the treatment plan according to a fixed time line, but for compliance with Joint Commission requirements, the organization must set the time frame for reviewing treatment plans. The rationale for reevaluating and revising the treatment plan goals and objectives is to ensure that the plan is monitored and updated so that individuals' progress can be measured and addressed. A discussion of integrating measurement-based care is provided in Chapter 3.

Challenges When Revising Plan Goals and Objectives

While on survey, a Joint Commission surveyor was reviewing an individual's treatment plan but found no evidence that the individual's plan had been reevaluated despite progress notes indicating that the individual said, "I am not doing well." Additional notes revealed the individual's concerns about his continued sobriety. In this case, progress notes over a three-month period included a note of intention to review and reevaluate the treatment plan, but there was no evidence of revised goals or objectives. In this particular situation, the Joint Commission surveyor would indicate that the BHC organization was not complying with the standards regarding reevaluation of goals and objectives. More importantly, it may be indicative of overall poor quality of care, treatment, and services at this BHC organization.

It should be noted that a review of the treatment plan may not necessarily result in changes to goals or objectives. It should be documented, however, that a review took place and why there was no change. For example, a physician may have started an individual on a new medication for which the dosage is being adjusted. The individual may continue to experience the problems the medication was prescribed to address. When the treatment plan is reviewed, it may be determined that the medication needs to continue to be titrated, but the schedule outlined for goals and objectives requires no change.

In another case, an organization's policy mandated weekly reviews of treatment plans to assess an individual's progress; however, a surveyor cited the organization for no reviews having occurred for a client who had been receiving services for two months. To ensure compliance, in the first example the individual's lack of progress warranted reevaluation of treatment, while in the second case the organization was cited for not following its own policies.

Deferred Goals

Reasons for deferral of a goal—or the objectives related to a goal—must also be included in the treatment plan. So far, this book has emphasized the importance of setting goals and objectives to reach those goals, so certainly if a goal is deferred—particularly, after all the effort to identify and set that goal—explanation and documentation is warranted in the individual's treatment plan. For example, if, during treatment planning, an individual shares that he would also like to work on improving his marriage but has identified his priority goal as managing his mental health condition, that relationship goal might be included in the treatment plan but flagged as deferred. The relationship goal could then be revisited during plan reviews to determine if the individual is ready to initiate interventions to meet the goal or later when a referral to a marriage counselor might be more appropriate. In addition, individuals may not want to work on trauma because it may trigger unpleasant symptoms. Deferring a goal may be necessary when trying to triage priorities of all goals, or when the individual served experiences a change in life circumstances, such as the unexpected loss of a job or loss of a loved one. An example of a prioritized goal may involve an individual who indicates a desire to stop smoking but is having symptoms of depression, causing her trouble getting out of bed each morning.

As a result, she is missing work or is repeatedly late for work. Her smoking is a coping strategy—albeit an unhealthy one—that helps her manage her depression. The clinician and the individual may together decide that it is of greater priority to manage the depression first, perhaps with medication and other strategies, and that smoking cessation should be a deferred goal. Frequently, organizations fail to document the reason a goal is deferred and may be cited for this on a Joint Commission survey. It is important to note that the rationale for goal deferral must be documented in the treatment plan. Refer to the sample treatment plans in Chapter 5 for an example of a deferred goal and the rationale behind it.

Including Interventions That Meet Identified Goals

After identifying the individual's needs, goals, strengths, and preferences, treatment interventions are developed and included in the treatment plan. **Interventions** are clinical tools used by the treatment team to help individuals achieve their goals and objectives. Interventions promote and inform the steps an individual can take to do something about undesirable or unhealthy behaviors. It is important to recognize that the intervention is not an end point; it is the means by which something specific and individualized to the person served is being addressed. It may take the form of group therapy to help an individual manage feelings of grief or loss. Interventions may also involve lifestyle changes, such as eating well and exercising to help combat depression. The actions taken are controlled by the individual, so it is important to ensure that the intervention helps the person served in an individualized way.

When developing planned interventions, consider the individual's preferences that were captured during screening and assessment, which may include the following:

- Preferred appointment times; for example, early morning, after lunch, late afternoon
- Location/method of treatment; for example, in-person, virtual, at school, in a group setting

Additional details about an individual's preferences may be formed by staff when staff ask the following:

- What interventions are likely to be most effective and support measurable progress?
- Based on the strengths of the individual, how frequently should the intervention(s) be implemented? At what intensity or duration? Daily interventions may be fine, but others may be weekly or even monthly.
- What skills does the individual have or need to effectively implement the interventions? For example, an individual may already practice yoga regularly at home, so that can be included as an intervention to prevent anxiety and stress.

The treatment plan should identify each intervention in precise language, staff responsibilities for each intervention, and the individual's response to the intervention. This is particularly important for interdisciplinary care in which effective coordination of care, treatment, or services depends on good communication and shared knowledge among staff. The following are some examples of clear interventions that involve interdisciplinary care that could be included in a treatment plan:

- Routine nutritional counseling and education in oral health for individuals with eating disorders
- Participation in social and community situations, such as an employment service that provides a job coach or mentor for individuals with intellectual and developmental disabilities.
- Provision of age-appropriate education for children or youth whose care, treatment, or services require a prolonged absence from school
- Medication(s) administered and reconciled logs for drugs prescribed in a methadone maintenance program

There may be multiple interventions for the same identified goal. For example, an individual may receive several services concurrently that include, for example, medication services, individual therapy, group therapy, and/or intensive case management. For each intervention—whether individual therapy, group therapy, or case management—responsible staff members must provide a specific description within the treatment plan of the service provided and its frequency. The description might include weekly, multiple times per week, or an increase and/or decrease as the individual progresses and/or regresses. Nonspecific frequency descriptors, such as "as needed" or "as appropriate," fail to meet language requirements and will likely be cited for noncompliance on a Joint Commission survey. Examples of multiple interventions may include the following:

- Therapist will provide individual therapy weekly for the next six months and use cognitive behavioral therapy (for example, learning to replace harmful thoughts with helpful ones) to improve mood and score on the PHQ-9 assessment tool.
- Group therapist will provide mindfulness techniques in weekly group therapy sessions for the next three months to help the individual reduce anxiety.
- Psychiatrist will manage medication one to eight times over the next three months to decrease anxiety.
- The case manager will collaborate with the treatment team, including psychiatrist, psychotherapist, and/or community support workers, one to four times per month to provide continuity of care.

A strategy for ensuring that the plan includes effective interventions is to review the individual's preferences that were captured as part of screening activities. Recall that an individuals' preferences include factors that help determine whether they will be engaged in their treatment and treatment planning. In other words, all the interventions in the world will not matter unless individuals indicate that they are able and willing to participate or engage in the interventions. These preferences may include culture or language preferences, for example, but may also include preferred coping strategies, such as listening to music, practicing meditation, or exercising. This information can be captured in discussions with the individual served or by using a self-report form that can be completed by the individual. Another strategy is to review outcomes measures, which are discussed in more detail in Chapter 3. An effective treatment plan should include measurements of outcomes as individuals progress toward achieving their identified goals.

Involving Family in the Plan

Many situations demand the need for family involvement during treatment planning. This is particularly true in cases in which the care, treatment, or service is for the welfare of a child (*see* Chapter 4). Insight from family members can also assist the care team in developing a treatment plan that the individual is more likely to engage in, and family may encourage goal accountability. Joint Commission Standard CTS.03.01.05, EP 1, requires that "the family of the individual served is involved in developing the plan for care, treatment, or services upon consent from the individual (if an adult) or in accordance with law and regulation (if a minor), unless such participation is contraindicated." Information gathered during screening and assessment should include insight into family member relations and whether family involvement is contraindicated due to substance abuse, violence, contributions to the individual's problem(s), or denial of the necessity for the individual's treatment. It may also indicate which family members may be better suited for such involvement and which should be excluded to improve outcomes.

Many BHC programs invite family to join sessions with the individual served to achieve this purpose. Often this is a part of their programming. With adults, family involvement may start with a Release of Information signed by the individual giving permission for participation in treatment. In such cases, family members may join in a therapy session with the individual served or participate in a family program without the individual served.

Family involvement in treatment planning can be beneficial and appropriate for many individuals, but there are some individuals for whom involvement of family is actually recommended. The following list is by no means exhaustive but does include individuals for whom family involvement is often appropriate and helpful to successful treatment:

- Individuals with eating disorders
- Individuals experiencing a recent traumatic event or post-traumatic stress disorder
- Individuals with severe mental health disorders
- Individuals with intellectual and developmental disabilities
- Individuals in substance use recovery programs
- Individuals recovering from abuse or neglect, provided the family member is not the perpetrator or enabler of the abuse or neglect and there is no legal action, such as a restraining order, in place that prohibits contact
- Individuals who have attempted or are at risk of suicide

Managing and Documenting a Referral

It is common for BHC organizations to refer individuals to alternative or additional resources for more specialized treatment if care, treatment, or services exceeds the organization's capabilities. Your organization's BHC's screening and assessment processes will indicate whether the individual's treatment falls within your facility's scope of service. If an individual needs additional care that is not offered by your organization (for example, an individual needs treatment for substance use disorder and your organization does not offer that service), a referral should be made and included in the individual's clinical or case record. Likewise, if a physical screening and assessment of medical history reveal an individual is pregnant and does not have an established obstetrician-gynecologist, your organization may refer that individual for obstetrical services. Treatment plans should reflect when individuals are receiving concurrent care, treatment, or services provided by an outside source that is integral to meeting their goals and objectives as part of the plan for care your organization provides.

However, even after developing a treatment plan, there may be situations when services may need to be delayed and a referral made to an alternate provider. For example, if an individual is receiving behavioral health care treatment, care, or services to manage an anxiety disorder and she begins to show signs of psychosis, but your facility does not provide services to individuals with severe mental health conditions, you must refer that individual to an appropriate provider. Finally, if an individual is not meeting planned treatment goals, and behaviors are not improving (for whatever reason), an offer to refer that individual to a provider who may provide alternative therapies outside your scope of service is appropriate. Joint Commission Standard CTS.03.01.07 requires that referrals be made and documented in the individual's clinical/case record whenever individuals need additional care, treatment, or services not offered by the organization.

Regarding an organization's expectations for documentation and following up on referrals made, a Joint Commission surveyor may look for documentation in the treatment plan review that the clinician engaged in discussion with an individual about follow-up on referrals made for alternative services. It should be noted in the treatment plan reviews.

Summary

As we continue to build the foundation for an effective individualized treatment plan, this chapter discussed gathering and applying assessment data in treatment planning to develop an individual's goals and objectives. This chapter also explored the significance of reassessing individuals and reevaluating the treatment plan throughout the course of treatment to monitor progress in care. Chapter 3 will explore integrating measurement-based care into treatment planning as a way to monitor both the individual's progress and the organization's improvement efforts.

Reference

1. Coulter A, Collins A. *Making Shared Decision-Making a Reality: No Decision About Me, Without Me*. London: The King's Fund, 2011. Accessed Dec 22, 2021. https://www.kingsfund.org.uk/sites/files/kf/Making-shared-decision-making-a-reality-paper-Angela-Coulter-Alf-Collins-July-2011_0.pdf.

Tool 2-1. Sample Patient Health Questionnaire-9 (PHQ-9) for Depression

DOWNLOAD

Date_______________Patient Name:______________________________Date of Birth: ____________

Over the last 2 weeks, how often have you been bothered by any of the following problems? Please circle your answers.

PHQ-9 Items	**Not at all**	**Several days**	**More than half the days**	**Nearly every day**
1. Little interest or pleasure in doing things.	0	1	2	3
2. Feeling down, depressed, or hopeless.	0	1	2	3
3. Trouble falling or staying asleep or sleeping too much.	0	1	2	3
4. Feeling tired or having little energy.	0	1	2	3
5. Poor appetite or overeating.	0	1	2	3
6. Feeling bad about yourself – or that you are a failure or have let yourself or your family down.	0	1	2	3
7. Trouble concentrating on things, such as reading the newspaper or watching television.	0	1	2	3
8. Moving or speaking so slowly that other people could have noticed. Or the opposite – being so fidgety or restless that you have been moving around a lot more than usual.	0	1	2	3
9. Thoughts that you would be better off dead, or of hurting yourself in some way.	0	1	2	3
Add the score for each column				

For Office Coding: __________ +________ + ____________+ __________

=Total Score: ____________

If you checked off any problems, how difficult have these problems made it for you to do your work, take care of things at home, or get along with other people? (Circle one):

Not difficult at all **Somewhat difficult** **Very difficult** **Extremely difficult**

Tool 2-2. Sample Generalized Anxiety Disorder-7 (GAD-7) Questionnaire

DOWNLOAD

Date_______________Patient Name:______________________________Date of Birth: ____________

Over the <u>last 2 weeks</u>, how often have you been bothered by any of the following problems? Please circle your answers.

GAD-7 Items	Not at all sure	Several days	Over half the days	Nearly every day
1. Feeling nervous, anxious, or on edge.	0	1	2	3
2. Not being able to stop or control worrying.	0	1	2	3
3. Worrying too much about different things.	0	1	2	3
4. Trouble relaxing.	0	1	2	3
5. Being so restless that it's hard to sit still.	0	1	2	3
6. Becoming easily annoyed or irritable.	0	1	2	3
7. Feeling afraid as if something awful might happen.	0	1	2	3
Add the score for each column				

Total Score (add your column scores): ____________

If you checked off <u>any</u> problems, how <u>difficult</u> have these problems made it for you to do your work, take care of things at home, or get along with other people? (Circle one):

Not difficult at all **Somewhat difficult** **Very difficult** **Extremely difficult**

Chapter 3
Integrating Measurement-Based Care in the Treatment Plan

Relevant Standards Covered in This Chapter	
CTS.03.01.09	The organization assesses the outcomes of care, treatment, or services provided to the individual served.
	EP 1 The organization uses a standardized tool or instrument to monitor the individual's progress in achieving the individual's care, treatment, or service goals. **Note:** Ideally, the tool or instrument monitors progress from the individual's perspective. The tool or instrument may be focused on a population or diagnostic category (such as depression or anxiety), or the tool or instrument may have a more global focus such as general distress, functional status, quality of life (especially in regard to intellectual/developmental disabilities and other physical and/or sensory disabilities), well-being, or permanency (especially in regard to foster care or other out-of-home care for children and youth).
	EP 2 The organization gathers and analyzes the data generated through standardized monitoring, and the results are used to inform the goals and objectives of the individual's plan for care, treatment, or services as needed.
	EP 3 The organization evaluates the outcomes of care, treatment, or services provided to the population(s) it serves by aggregating and analyzing the data gathered through the standardized monitoring effort. (For more information, refer to Standard PI.02.01.01) (*See also* LD.03.07.01, EP 2)
	EP 4 For organizations that provide eating disorders care, treatment, or services: The organization assesses outcomes of care, treatment, or services based on data collected at admission. Examples of such data include complete history and physical including height, weight, frequency of binge eating and purging (when applicable), eating disorder diagnosis, body mass index (BMI), heart rate, date of last period, and other appropriate lab tests such as potassium, phosphorus, thyroid, hemoglobin, glucose, as determined by the organization and in accordance with the level of care provided. (*See also* CTS.02.03.11, EP 1)

Relevant Standards Covered in This Chapter	
LD.03.07.01	Leaders establish priorities for performance improvement. (Refer to the "Performance Improvement" [PI] chapter.)
	EP 2 As part of performance improvement, leaders do the following: • Set priorities for performance improvement activities and care, treatment, or service outcomes for individuals served • Give priority to high-volume, high-risk, or problem-prone processes for improvement activities • Identify the frequency of data collection for performance improvement activities • Reprioritize performance improvement activities in response to changes in the internal or external environment **Note 1:** For child welfare agencies, patient health outcomes for children and youth might include placement in permanent family homes, long-term functional outcomes, contact with family members, parent satisfaction, child and youth satisfaction, and foster parent satisfaction. **Note 2:** For child welfare agencies, examples of high-volume, high-risk, or problem-prone processes include multiple placements (placement instability), elopement/runaway, and aggressive/violent behaviors. (*See also* CTS.03.01.09, EP 3; PI.01.01.01, EPs 1, 2, 12, 13, 20; PI.02.01.01, EP 1)
PI.03.01.01	The organization compiles and analyzes data.
	EP 8 The organization uses the results of data analysis to identify improvement opportunities. (*See also* CTS.02.04.25, EP 7; HRM.01.06.05, EP 2; HRM.01.07.01, EP 3)

Note: Joint Commission standards are updated on a regular basis. Always refer to the most current version of the *Comprehensive Accreditation Manual for Behavioral Health Care and Human Services* (*CAMBHC*) or its E-dition® counterpart for requirements relevant to your setting.

Terms to Know

aggregate data
data management
measurement-based care
Patient Health Questionnaire-9 (PHQ-9)

Introduction

In 2018 The Joint Commission revised the outcomes of Care, Treatment, and Services (CTS) Standard CTS.03.01.09 for accredited behavioral health care and human services (BHC) organizations to add the use of a standardized tool or instrument to assess outcomes of care.[1] The revised standard also requires that accredited organizations use the data gathered to monitor the individual's progress, inform the individual's goals and objectives, and drive decisions about care. This is a process known as **measurement-based care** (sometimes referred to as feedback-informed treatment, outcome-informed care, or other names). There is now more than 20 years of research that supports measurement-based care as improving the outcomes of behavioral health care, treatment, and services. These findings are robust, and they extend across a broad range of modalities, populations, and settings. These include individual psychotherapy, couples and family therapy, group therapy, substance use treatment, eating disorder programs, pharmacological treatment, services for children and adolescents, and settings as diverse as outdoor/wilderness facilities and community mental health care settings. When successfully implemented, measurement-based care benefits both individuals served and the BHC organizations that provide care, treatment, or services to them. When organizations establish policies and procedures for developing treatment plans, they can incorporate collecting and using data from standardized outcome tools to set goals and capture progress for each individual served.

Criteria for Selecting a Measurement-Based Tool

There are many tools and instruments available to monitor and assess an individual's progress toward achieving goals and outcomes of care. As mentioned in previous chapters, The Joint Commission does not prescribe the use of any particular tools, but it does specify in CTS.03.01.09, Element of Performance (EP) 1, that the tool or instrument chosen be standardized and that it monitor progress of the individual served. Effective tools should be reliable, validated, and evidence based, and the outcomes evaluated by the tool should be consistent with the objectives of services. Chosen tools may focus on a diagnostic category—such as depression or anxiety—if services are intended to address these diagnostic categories. In some cases, however, tools may have a broad focus, such as the following:

- General distress
- Functional status
- Quality of life
- Well-being
- Permanency (for foster care or out-of-home care for children and youth)

The key is for organizations to choose standardized instruments appropriate for the population served. This is critical to provide meaningful results related to the individual's treatment goals. For a tool to comply with the Joint Commission requirements, it must meet the following criteria:

- Have well-established psychometric properties (reliability and validity). Appropriate instruments should have been tested for their reliability (consistency as a measure) and validity (measuring what they are intending to measure). Results of this testing will likely be published. Organizations are encouraged to learn about the instrument's reliability and validity as they weigh their options for standardized tools. This can be done by evaluating benchmark data and published results of psychometric testing, and also by examining the research on how widely used the instrument is and under which circumstances and settings it has proven most effective.
- Documented sensitivity to change (that is, the ability to detect true and meaningful changes over time). Instruments that include a "reliable change index" or similar construct can be used to distinguish statistically significant or meaningful changes from normal or expected variation. When determining the impact of care, it is critical to distinguish between changes that represent true improvement or deterioration versus typical variations that might be expected on a daily, weekly, or monthly basis. Staff should be trained to understand a typical variation in data. For example, although a one- or two-point difference in scores on the depression scale may be attributed to minor variations between administrations, a five-point change is clinically significant.
- Used as a repeated measure (the instrument or tool is designed to be administered at multiple intervals for the purpose of detecting change over time). Instruments, such as the **Patient Health Questionnaire-9 (PHQ-9)**, which can be used for routine outcome measures for depression, are meant to be administered repeatedly. The frequency of use is an important consideration for organizations and is based on the types and typical lengths of services they provide. The organization should select a tool or instrument that can be administered frequently enough to ensure that the care the individual is receiving can be adjusted (when and if necessary). The frequency of administration of the tool depends on the tool itself and its intended use. (A caveat: Although not a Joint Commission requirement, a good practice is to align the frequency of tool administration with treatment plan review and document the individual's score each time to provide a data point as evidence that the individual is either progressing or regressing.)
- Established norms. Depending on setting and population served, an individuals' scores on an instrument should indicate their current state relative to a norm or benchmark (for example, responses to questions using the PHQ-9 assessment tool provide an indication of an individual's level of depression). Organizations are required to use tools that are appropriate and applicable to the individuals served.

The PHQ-9, which is one of the validated, evidence-based tools listed in Table 1-1 and also discussed in Chapter 2, is frequently used for assessing progress in an individual treated for depression. Application of this tool in practice is discussed in more detail below and in a sample treatment plan in Chapter 5.

Monitoring the Individual's Progress

As we've established, the expressed goals of an individual provide a contextual framework for data collected during screening and assessment and, as a result, drive the plan of care. By definition, a treatment plan must include a general outline of prescribed treatment, but it must also include measurements of outcomes as individuals progress toward achieving their identified goals. Feedback from screening and assessment tools can help organizations with setting goals, monitoring individuals' progress, and decision making when planning treatment and interventions.

The PHQ-9, a sample of which is included in Chapter 2, is an instrument used for individuals with depressive disorders. When properly used, it complies with Joint Commission requirements. The PHQ-9 consists of nine questions designed to assess an individual's level of depression. Each response is scored from 0 to 3, with a total score range from 0 to 27. Specific ranges of scores reflect varying levels of depression severity (for example, scores from 5 to 9 indicate mild depression, whereas scores from 20 to 27 indicate severe depression). Table 3-1 provides diagnosis and proposed treatment based on an individual's PHQ-9 score.

During initial contact with an individual, an organization may choose to administer the PHQ-9 as part of its screening and assessment processes. The PHQ-9 can be administered at admission, during treatment planning, throughout the course of treatment, and at discharge. For example, based on the interpretation of an individual's PHQ-9 score during intake, if an individual receives a total score of 21, treatment would be implemented that aligns with recommendations for individuals in the range of severe depression.

After discussion with the individual, a treatment plan would be developed that includes goals and objectives designed to reduce symptoms of depression. Interventions may include cognitive behavioral therapy through daily counseling sessions, among others. Goals may take into consideration the individual's intake PHQ-9 score and include measurable objectives for improvement, such as "to score 15 or lower on the PHQ-9 scale when administered again." After five sessions, the PHQ-9 is administered again, and the individual's score has declined to 12, or moderate depression. At this point, the treatment plan might be modified to reduce the frequency of counseling sessions, for example. However, after 10 sessions, the PHQ-9 is administered again, and the individual receives a score of 19, which indicates moderately severe depression. Based on these data, the clinician might discuss with the individual this change in score and whether—and to what degree—it may be necessary to modify the treatment plan to address the change in assessment status. Such a scenario serves to exemplify how data from this or other tools can be used to both monitor an individual's progress toward goals and to prompt adjustments in an individual's treatment plan.

Organizations are encouraged to share data from such tools with the individual served as part of the individual's treatment. It can be beneficial to graphically display results as a means of providing ongoing feedback to monitor clinical progress or lack thereof. For example, individuals may believe they are not making

Table 3-1. Interpretation of PHQ-9 Assessment Score

PHQ-9 Score	Depression Severity	Proposed Treatment
0–4	None–minimal	None
5–9	Mild	Watchful waiting; repeat PHQ-9 at follow-up
10–14	Moderate	Treatment plan: consider counseling, follow-up, and/or pharmacotherapy
15–19	Moderately severe	Active treatment with pharmacotherapy and/or psychotherapy
20–27	Severe	Immediate initiation of pharmacotherapy and, if severe impairment or poor response to therapy, expedited referral to a mental health specialist for psychotherapy and/or collaborative management

much progress, whereas an objective measurement tool may indicate otherwise. Conversely, an individual served (or a clinician) may overestimate progress. Sharing objective results can move an individual toward a more realistic understanding of progress.

Monitoring the Organization's Progress

A BHC organization and its performance improvement staff may use **aggregate data** from such measurement-based outcome tools to drive organizational improvement efforts and to evaluate efficacy of the interventions provided to populations served. For example, such aggregate data can reveal improvements in symptoms and/or functioning at discharge or throughout stages of treatment or services. Aggregate data from the PHQ-9 tool, for example, may show that improvement outcomes of individuals diagnosed with depression were lower than the organization anticipated in 10 weeks after 10 individual sessions.

The organization may then take a closer look at outcome data, perhaps by using a satisfaction survey, and discover a common theme: Many individuals felt socially isolated and would have preferred to share experiences with others for support and ideas. As a result, the organization may add an open process therapy group and find that when aggregate outcome data are analyzed again, average improvements at 10 weeks increased significantly.

A rationale for this standard is to encourage organizations to continuously strive to improve the quality of their processes to ensure better outcomes for individuals served. Organizations should not only have a policy or procedure for using standardized tools to monitor outcomes of care but must also understand the process and rationale for gathering data as a means to improve their services. Tool 3-1 on page 58 is a sample template designed to help organizations develop measurement policies and procedures for using standardized outcome tools to monitor the progress of individuals served.

Other Measurement-Based Instruments

Some BHC organizations' stakeholders, including regulators, may identify and mandate certain measurement tools. To comply with Joint Commission requirements, organizations must verify that those mandated tools also meet The Joint Commission's criteria for measurement-based care and are used appropriately. The Joint Commission offers on its website a Behavioral Healthcare Instruments Listing that includes dozens of measurement-based care tools and instruments.[2] The instruments listing is a resource, and tool developers are encouraged to visit the listings page and share their measurement-based care instruments. The Joint Commission does not endorse any particular instruments in the listing, nor does it imply that the list is exhaustive. Some tools are proprietary and require a paid subscription for use from the developer, whereas others are in the public domain and free to use. Organizations may use this searchable resource to identify measurement tools based on their needs and the needs of the individuals they serve. Each tool listed includes details about its appropriate use, relevant population, program setting, benchmark data, and psychometric testing for validity and reliability.

In addition, *A Core Set of Outcomes Measures for Behavioral Health Across Service Settings*, an issue brief developed by the Kennedy Forum, addresses evidence-based measures and how they can be integrated and applied across an organization to support measurement-based care.[3] The issue brief offers guidance on integrating measurement-based care when planning treatment for behavioral health conditions. It also provides validated clinical rating scales that can be applied across multiple health sectors—including specialty behavioral health care—that support standardized assessment and clinical decision making. This core set of outcome measures is meant to encourage systemwide, measurement-based care in treating behavioral health conditions that will help providers determine whether the treatment plan is working and help facilitate treatment adjustments, consultations, or referrals for higher-intensity services when individuals are not improving as expected.

Factors to Consider for Compliance

BHC organizations should always consider what works for their needs, budget, and technical requirements when choosing measurement tools and instruments. Staff may require specialized training and education to use and interpret a tool. Staff training on the use and benefit of measurement tools cannot be overlooked.

Joint Commission surveyors have reported that although some organizations have integrated tools in their practice, they have not trained staff to use them as intended. Often staff feel as though the tool is simply an administrative task and fail to see the tool's value in verifying whether interventions are working. Some tools require licensing. Electronic medical records programs frequently have built-in measurement tools that can be used for compliance, provided they fit the criteria for a standardized tool.

Using a standardized instrument or tool is an important step, but the act alone is not sufficient for compliance with Standard CTS.03.01.09. The standard requires that organizations use data gathered from the instrument to monitor an individual's progress and to inform care, treatment, or services. However, over the past five years, this requirement was scored for noncompliance on nearly half of all BHC surveys. If an organization has not selected an instrument, is not consistently administering the instrument selected, or is using the instrument only at intake and discharge, surveyors will cite the organization for noncompliance under EP 2: *The organization gathers and analyzes the data generated through standardized monitoring, and the results are used to inform the goals and objectives of the individual's plan for care, treatment, or services as needed.*

Organizations must collect data throughout the care process; otherwise, they are not using data to assess progress while the individual is engaged in care. This is often easy for Joint Commission surveyors to observe during the survey and through conversations with providers about what data are being used to monitor the individual's progress and inform care. Tools, when used properly, provide guidance on what is considered progress. A good practice is for organizations to graph data collected from tools to show the trends and visually highlight an individual's progress at each treatment plan review to determine whether data reflect the service provided.

BHC organizations also struggle to comply because measurement-based care is a cultural shift. Some providers have not worked with objective data, and interpreting and effectively using data may be foreign and uncomfortable. Practical challenges associated with implementing measurement-based care include building a consistent and efficient process for collecting measurement-based care data, delivering feedback to providers, creating workflows that make data readily available, and building processes to aggregate data. All these challenges require commitment from leadership, time, resources, and effective change management.

Assessing Data Management

To enhance performance and evaluate organizational practices related to measurement-based care, BHC organizations should also perform **data management** reviews. BHC organizations can use outcome measurement tracer questions to assess how they analyze and aggregate data to identify opportunities for improvement. Tool 3-2 on page 62 provides some outcome measurement tracer questions to explore how data are collected, analyzed, aggregated, and managed in your organization.

Using Data for Quality and Performance Improvement

Organizations can also use aggregate data to inform quality improvement efforts. In some organizations, members of the Care, Treatment, and Services Committee may collaborate with the Performance Improvement Committee to collect and analyze data as part of the organization's established improvement activities.

Entering data into a spreadsheet and tracking performance on a graph is only a small part of effective quality improvement. The goal of standard CTS.03.01.09—consistent with the general quality improvement mission of The Joint Commission—is to use data collected to explore opportunities to provide higher-quality care, treatment, or services. In the aggregate, the data from standardized tools and instruments can identify specific programs, service areas, units, or practitioners that could benefit from additional resources or education (or to identify exceptional performers who can mentor others or take on the most difficult cases).[4–6] Organizations may also choose to use aggregate data to demonstrate the value they provide to the individuals and populations they serve by illustrating improvements.

Summary

This chapter emphasizes the importance of adopting measurement- (or outcomes)-based care to simultaneously monitor individuals' progress and response to treatment, as well as to identify opportunities for improvement and add value to the services they provide. Integrating standardized assessment data into care planning from the start can show the impact of treatment on individuals served. When the organization and the individual served can objectively see actual measured outcomes of care, it informs shared decision making about whether to stay the course or make corrections. This leads to positive outcomes, which results in higher-quality care, treatment, and services.

References

1. The Joint Commission. Revised outcome measures standard for behavioral health care. *R^3 Report*, Issue 13. Feb 6, 2018. Accessed Dec 23, 2021. https://www.jointcommission.org/standards/r3-report/r3-report-issue-13-revised-outcome-measures-standard-for-behavioral-health-care/.

2. The Joint Commission. Behavioral Healthcare Instruments Listing. Accessed Dec 23, 2021. https://manual.jointcommission.org/BHCInstruments/WebHome.?_ga=2.195810922.713509994.1619106682-1490815834.1618759591.

3. The Kennedy Forum. *A Core Set of Outcome Measures for Behavioral Health Across Service Settings*. Issue Brief. 2015. Accessed Dec 23, 2021. http://www.thekennedyforum.org/app/uploads/2020/02/MBC_supplement.pdf.

4. Duncan BL. *On Becoming a Better Therapist: Evidence-Based Practice One Client at a Time*, 2nd ed. Washington, DC: American Psychological Association, 2014.

5. Chow DL, et al. The role of deliberate practice in the development of highly effective psychotherapists. *Psychotherapy* (Chic). 2015 Sep;52(3):337–345

6. Miller SD, et al. Making treatment count: Client-directed, outcome-informed clinical work with problem drinkers. *Psychotherapy in Australia*. 2005;11(4):42–56.

Tool 3-1. Sample Outcomes of Care, Treatment, or Services Measurement Procedures Policy Template

DOWNLOAD

Tool 3-1. Sample Outcomes of Care, Treatment, or Services Measurement Procedures Policy Template

[Logo]	**TITLE** Outcomes of Care, Treatment, or Services Measurement Procedures		**IDENTIFICATION NUMBER** [Number]
ORGANIZATION(S) [Organization]	**LEVEL** ☐ System ☐ Organization ☐ Division ☐ Department	**CATEGORY** ☐ Clinical ☐ Management ☐ Regulatory	**POSTING DATE** [MM/DD/YYYY] **EFFECTIVE DATE** [MM/DD/YYYY]
REVIEW CYCLE ☐ 1 year ☐ 3 years **LAST REVIEW DATE:** [MM/DD/YYYY]		**REPLACES** **TITLE:** Outcomes of Care, Treatment, or Services Measurement Procedures **EFFECTIVE DATE(S):** [MM/DD/YYYY]	

PROCEDURES STATEMENT
The progress of each individual served is monitored using standardized outcome tools.

PURPOSE
To establish procedures for using standardized outcome tools to monitor the progress of individuals served and the outcomes of their care, treatment, or services to continuously improve the quality and safety of the care, treatment, or services provided by the organization.

SCOPE
Applies to all care, treatment, or services provided by the organization.

Applies to all areas of the organization that participate in the care, treatment, or services of individuals served.

Applies to all staff members who participate in care, treatment, or services of individuals served.

Applies to all individuals who receive care, treatment, or services from the organization.

DEFINITIONS
Adult – An individual who has reached the age of legal majority.

Assessment – 1. The process established by the organization for obtaining clinically relevant information about each individual seeking behavioral health care, treatment, or services. The information is used to match an individual's need with the appropriate setting, service/program, and intervention. 2. For opioid treatment programs, the process of identifying the precise nature and extent of a patient's substance use disorder and other medical, mental health, and social problems as a basis for treatment planning.

Child – A person between 0 and 12 years of age, or as determined by applicable law and regulation.

History and physical – Information gathered about an individual using a holistic approach for the purpose of establishing a diagnosis and developing a plan for care, treatment, or services to address physical health issues. The history may include information about previous illnesses; previous medical or surgical interventions and response to treatment; family health history; and social, cultural, economic, and lifestyle issues that may affect the individual's health and well-being. The physical involves the physical examination of the individual's body by the following means:

inspection, palpation, percussion, and auscultation. When used in concert with behavioral health care services, the history and physical may be used to rule out physical causes for behavioral health conditions or to assess the impact of a medical diagnosis or treatment on a behavioral health condition.

Medical history – A record consisting of an account of an individual's physical health history, obtained whenever possible from the individual, and including at least the following information: chief complaint, details of the present illness or care needs, relevant past history, and relevant inventory by body systems.

Outcome – A measure(s) that indicates the result of the care, treatment, or services provided.

Plan of care, treatment, or services – A written plan, based on data gathered during screening or assessment, that identifies care, treatment, or service needs, strengths, preferences, and goals; describes the strategy for meeting those needs, preferences, and goals; builds on the strengths and considers the preferences of the individuals served; and documents progress toward meeting the plan's objectives. The plan may include care, treatment, habilitation, and rehabilitation.

Reassessment – Ongoing data collection, which begins on initial assessment, comparing the most recent data with the data collected at earlier assessments.

Standardized outcome tool – A tool used to measure the outcomes of care, treatment, or services through measurement of the progress of the individual served. A strong outcome tool has the following components:

- Well-established psychometric properties (reliability and validity)
- Documented sensitivity to change (the ability to detect true or meaningful changes over time)
- Use as a repeated measure (can reliably detect change from administration to administration)
- Established norms (can distinguish between populations that need or do not need services)

Youth – A person 13 years of age or older who has not reached the age of majority, or as identified by law and regulation.

Responsibilities

The Care, Treatment, and Services (CTS) Committee is responsible for the following:

- Overseeing, reviewing, revising, maintaining, and implementing this policy
- In collaboration with the Performance Improvement Committee, collecting and analyzing data in compliance with this policy

Qualified staff are responsible for performing assessments and reassessments and documenting progress and outcomes.

All staff members who participate in an individual's care, treatment, or services are responsible for creating and maintaining that individual's plan of care, treatment, or services.

The Performance Improvement Committee is responsible for aggregating and analyzing data on the progress and outcomes of the population served, as part of its established improvement activities.

Procedures

Qualified staff members do the following:

1. Perform screenings, assessments, and reassessments of the individual served, as described in organization policy.
2. Engage the patient and, if appropriate, family members in performing all assessments and reassessments, whenever possible.

3. Create a plan of care, treatment, or services for the individual served, as described in organization policy.
4. Determine standardized outcome tool(s) that are appropriate for assessing the progress of the individual served, based on factors including, but not limited to, the following:
    - Age, gender, or other population data
    - Diagnostic category
    - Global issues applicable to the care, treatment, or services provided, such as functional status, quality of life, well-being, or permanency
5. Use the information gathered from the standardized outcome tool(s) to inform decisions about the individual's plan of care, treatment, or services, in collaboration with individuals and/or their family, as appropriate. (Note: More than one tool may be used based on the population served.) These decisions include, but are not limited to, the following:
    - Goals of care, treatment, or services
    - Objectives to achieving stated goals
6. Use the appropriate standardized outcome tool(s) to assess and document the individuals' progress in achieving his or her documented goals.
7. Record the outcomes from the perspective of individuals served using their own words, whenever possible.
8. Perform these processes at the following times:
    - At admission
    - During the course of treatment, as applicable
    - Whenever the individual's plan of care, treatment, or services is revised
    - At discharge or transfer
9. Collaborate with the Performance Improvement Committee and its data aggregation and analysis activities, as appropriate.

PROCEDURES FOR ORGANIZATIONS THAT PROVIDE CARE, TREATMENT, OR SERVICES FOR INDIVIDUALS WITH EATING DISORDERS

Qualified staff do the following:

1. Use appropriate standardized outcome tools to collect data on the individual's physical health.
2. Include at least the following elements, as applicable to the individual:
    - Height
    - Weight
    - Frequency of binge eating and purging
    - Eating disorder diagnosis
    - Body mass index (BMI)
    - Heart rate
    - Date of last period
    - Lab test results (for example, potassium, phosphorus, thyroid, hemoglobin, glucose)
    - Other elements identified by the organization
3. Collect these data at the following times:
    - At admission
    - During the course of treatment, as applicable
    - Whenever the individual's plan of care, treatment, or services is revised
    - At discharge or transfer
4. Use these data collected at admission to assess outcomes of care, treatment, or services.

References

Joint Commission Standard CTS.03.01.09, Element of Performance (EP) 1. The organization uses a standardized tool or instrument to monitor the individual's progress in achieving the individual's care, treatment, or service goals.

Joint Commission Standard CTS.03.01.09, EP 2. The organization gathers and analyzes the data generated through standardized monitoring, and the results are used to inform the goals and objectives of the individual's plan for care, treatment, or services as needed.

Joint Commission Standard CTS.03.01.09, EP 3. The organization evaluates the outcomes of care, treatment, or services provided to the population(s) it serves by aggregating and analyzing the data gathered through the standardized monitoring effort. (For more information, refer to Standard PI.02.01.01).

Joint Commission Standard CTS.03.01.09, EP 4. **For organizations that provide eating disorders care, treatment, or services:** The organization assesses outcomes of care, treatment, or services based on data collected at admission. Examples of such data include complete history and physical including height, weight, frequency of binge eating and purging (when applicable), eating disorder diagnosis, body mass index (BMI), heart rate, date of last period, and other appropriate lab tests such as potassium, phosphorus, thyroid, hemoglobin, glucose, as determined by the organization and in accordance with the level of care provided.

Companion Policies

Discharge Planning Policy
Performance Improvement Plan
Plan for Care, Treatment, or Services Development Policy
Screening, Assessment, and Reassessment Policy

Approval

Name and Credentials [Name and Credentials] **Title** [Title]	**Name and Credentials** [Name and Credentials] **Title** [Title]
Signature	**Date** [MM/DD/YYYY]
Signature	**Date** [MM/DD/YYYY]

Tool 3-2. Sample Outcome Measurement Tracer Questions

DOWNLOAD

Tool 3-2. Sample Outcome Measurement Tracer Questions *You can use these sample questions for your mock tracers, adapting them as appropriate. Relevant standards cited are not necessarily applicable to every question.* *NOTE: The term* individual served *is used here to describe a recipient of care, treatment, or services. It can be replaced with the appropriate term for your accreditation program/setting.*
Relevant Standards: CTS.03.01.09, HRM.01.02.01, HRM.01.05.01, IM.01.01.01, IM.02.02.01, IM.02.02.03, LD.03.02.01, PI.01.01.01, PI.03.01.01
What is your approach to screening and assessment data use? Please describe your systems to collect, aggregate, analyze, and manage your data.
Who is responsible for overseeing your data management system? How is the system generally monitored and managed by the program?
When there are changes to be made to the plan of care, who is involved in that process and how are those changes documented?
What standardized instrument(s) or tool(s) does the organization use to assess and monitor progress throughout the care process?
How is the instrument(s) or tool(s) scored?
How often are outcome-based measurement tools readministered to monitor an individual's progress?
How do you use the data from these tools to inform the individual's care plan?
How is feedback from the instrument or tool delivered to members of the care team?
Is the individual served engaged and educated about these tools and the data collected?
How are scores and/or changes in scores discussed with the individual served?
Before selecting outcome-based measurement tools, how did you evaluate their psychometric qualities?
How did you determine their appropriateness for your setting?
How have staff been educated, trained, and supported to use these tools?
What process of aggregation and analysis is used to evaluate the outcomes for the populations served by the organization?
To what degree are the data used to assess change or improvement over time?
To what degree are the data used to assess individual clinician performance, unit or program performance, or effectiveness of services?
What electronic- and/or paper-based approaches do you have in place to collect data? How is this looked at for both care planning and outcome-based measurement purposes?
What outcome measures should you be measuring and reporting?
Please describe your initial assessment process for individuals who are new to the program. How is data management incorporated into this process?

Page **1** of **1**

Chapter 4
Planning for Unique Treatment Settings and Services

Relevant Standards Covered in This Chapter	
CTS.02.02.09	The organization has a process to provide medical histories, physical examinations, and diagnostic and laboratory tests.
	EP 5 For organizations providing care, treatment, or services to individuals with addictions: The program collects toxicological specimens in a manner that demonstrates trust and respect while taking reasonable steps to prevent falsification of samples. **Note:** Direct observation, although necessary for some individuals, is neither necessary nor appropriate for all individuals.
CTS.02.03.07	**For organizations providing care, treatment, or services to individuals with addictions:** The assessment includes the individual's history of addictive behaviors.
	EP 1 For organizations providing care, treatment, or services to individuals with addictions: The organization obtains the individual's history of alcohol use, drug use, nicotine use, and other addictive behaviors. The history includes the following information: • Age of onset • Method of acquiring substance • Duration • Patterns of use (for example, continuous, episodic, binge) • Frequency, amounts, and route of the substance that is taken
	EP 2 For organizations providing care, treatment, or services to individuals with addictions: The organization obtains the following information: • The individual's history of mental, emotional, behavioral, legal, and social consequences of dependence or addiction (for example, legal problems, divorce, loss of family members or friends, job-related incidents, financial difficulties, blackouts, memory impairment) • The individual's history of physical problems associated with substance abuse, dependence, and other addictive behaviors • History of the use of alcohol and other drugs and other addictive behaviors by the individual's family • If applicable to the belief system of the individual served, the individual's perception of the role of spirituality or religion in their life and recovery • The individual's readiness to change • The individual's current living arrangements and environment, and options for an alternative and supportive living environment

Relevant Standards Covered in This Chapter	
	EP 7 For organizations providing care, treatment, or services to individuals with addictions: Assessments of the individual served contain information about the following: • Previous care, treatment, or services • The individual's response to previous care, treatment, or services • The individual's relapse history • Acute intoxication and/or withdrawal potential
CTS.02.03.13	**For organizations providing care, treatment, or services to individuals with addictions:** The individual served is placed in the appropriate level of care.
	EP 1 For organizations providing care, treatment, or services to individuals with addictions: The organization uses an evidence-based, multidimensional admission assessment that includes, at a minimum, mental health, medical, and substance-use history for placement of the individual at the appropriate level of care.
CTS.02.03.15	**For organizations providing care, treatment, or services to individuals with addictions:** The organization uses drug testing to promote safety and quality of care.
	EP 1 For organizations providing care, treatment, or services to individuals with addictions: The organization follows its written policy on performing drug testing. **Note:** When developing this policy, the organization considers when drug testing is appropriate based on the individual's diagnosis, progress in treatment, history of use, and the provider's clinical judgment.
	EP 2 For organizations providing care, treatment, or services to individuals with addictions: The organization documents in the individual's clinical/case record the reason for drug testing, the results, and actions based on the results.
	EP 3 For organizations providing care, treatment, or services to individuals with addictions: The organization provides education and training for staff who are involved in drug testing. At a minimum, this includes test administration and storage of the specimen.
CTS.02.04.01	**For child welfare:** The agency screens and assesses each individual to determine needed services and/or placement.
	EP 18 For child welfare: The assessment is trauma-informed. **Note:** This should include the caregiver and/or parent's history of trauma as well as the individual served.
CTS.03.01.03	The organization has a plan for care, treatment, or services that reflects the assessed needs, strengths, preferences, and goals of the individual served.
	EP 28 For organizations providing care, treatment, or services to individuals with addictions: The organization develops a plan for care, treatment, or services at the time of admission or entry into care that reflects the assessed needs, strengths, preferences, and goals of the individual served.
CTS.03.02.03	**For child welfare:** The agency develops and periodically reviews its case plans.
	EP 1 For child welfare: The agency develops a case plan for each individual served.
	EP 2 For child welfare: The case plan is individualized based on an assessment of the emotional, behavioral, developmental, educational, spiritual, social, physical, cultural, linguistic, and legal status of the individual served as well as that of the family of origin.
	EP 3 For child welfare: When creating the case plan, the agency and family discuss potential triggering behaviors or conditions, as well as risk and protective factors, that led to abuse and neglect. In addition, the agency and family discuss the community resources that are available to alleviate the effects of maltreatment and prevent future incidents.

Relevant Standards Covered in This Chapter	
	EP 4 For child welfare: The case plan identifies the permanency goal if the individual is a child or youth in an out-of-home placement or foster care. This goal considers input from all parties and is reviewed according to law and regulation.
	EP 5 For child welfare: The case plan includes, at a minimum, short- and long-term goals, arrangement of services, sources of support, how the agency will help the family transition, and how it will advocate on the family's behalf.
	EP 6 For child welfare: The case plan addresses goals the family is expected to meet in a desired time frame and how the agency will help the family meet these goals.
	EP 7 For child welfare: The case planning process includes an assessment of preparation for transitional living when older youth or adults are discharged from foster care. (For more information on young adults preparing for transitional living, see Standard CTS.06.03.01) **Note:** Examples of activities that would help older youth or adults develop skills necessary for independence include the following: • Employment career planning assessments • Financial management • Daily living skills (for example, cooking, transportation) • Completing high school, general educational development (GED), or college • Job search training • Vocational training • Parenting skills • Developing social/relationship skills and support systems
	EP 8 For child welfare: When the agency has custody of the individual in foster care, the agency is responsible for case planning.
	EP 9 For child welfare: If the county or state agency retains custody and is responsible for the case plan, the child welfare agency participates in developing and evaluating the plan.
	EP 10 For child welfare: The case plan includes assessing potential reunification or other potential permanency options. If reunification is not possible, the plan includes counseling the family of origin about relinquishment and alternative placements. **Note:** If reunification is possible, it is the preferred goal.
	EP 11 For child welfare: The case plan includes an after-care plan that the agency must follow up with as appropriate or refer to the appropriate agencies and support for follow-up.
	EP 12 For child welfare: The agency has resources in place that identify support systems for youth as they transition to adulthood.
	EP 13 For child welfare: The agency evaluates the case plan in a time frame that is in accordance with organization policy and law and regulation.
	EP 14 For child welfare: The agency involves relevant persons in evaluating the case plan. **Note:** These persons may include agency staff, cross-sector contacts, the individual served, the foster parent(s), the family of origin (for children and youth only), and the representative of the state authority.
	EP 15 For child welfare: To promote the well-being of the child, care, treatment, or services in the home should be developmentally appropriate and supportive of the following: • Hygiene • Social interaction • Nutrition • Forming positive relationships • Education
	EP 16 For child welfare: The agency refers children to appropriate mental health services when the need is identified.

Relevant Standards Covered in This Chapter	
	EP 17 For child welfare: The agency, individual served, and family regularly review the case plan to assess progress. When needed, the case plan is adjusted to help the family continue to meet its goals.
HRM.01.05.01	Staff participate in education and training.
HRM.01.06.01	Staff are competent to perform their job duties and responsibilities.
	EP 7 For child welfare: Staff demonstrate cultural and age-specific competence.
LD.04.02.03	Ethical principles guide the organization's business practices.
	EP 10 For organizations providing care, treatment, or services to individuals with addictions: Prior to admission, information regarding charges and financial responsibility for care, treatment, or services are provided to the individual served. This includes making the individual aware of any travel or other expenses they will be responsible for related to the care, treatment, or services that the organization provides.

Note: Joint Commission standards are updated on a regular basis. Always refer to the most current version of the *Comprehensive Accreditation Manual for Behavioral Health Care and Human Services* (*CAMBHC*) or its E-dition® counterpart for requirements relevant to your setting.

Terms to Know

addiction services
case management, or coordination
case plan
child welfare agency
intensive outpatient program (IOP)
multidimensional assessment
permanency planning
resource family/parent
trauma-informed care

Introduction

The Joint Commission accredits many types of organizations under its Behavioral Health Care and Human Services (BHC) program. BHC–accredited organizations may serve individuals throughout their life span, for chronic conditions, or for a limited time to address acute conditions. BHC organizations may specialize in an age-related or special population group. They also operate in a variety of settings from facility based to community based. These variables (populations served, programs and services offered, and settings in which an organization operates) determine which Joint Commission standards and elements of performance (EPs) apply to your organization. This book has focused primarily on Joint Commission requirements in its "Care, Treatment, and Services" (CTS) chapter of the *Comprehensive Accreditation Manual for Behavioral Health Care and Human Services* (*CAMBHC*). This chapter includes the following:

- Standards that apply to all BHC settings
- Standards that apply to specific programs/services
- Standards that apply to specific populations with unique needs, including the following:
  - Individuals with addictions
  - Children/youth, including children receiving child welfare services*
  - Individuals with eating disorders
  - Individuals with intellectual and developmental disabilities

This chapter addresses specific, additional treatment planning requirements for individuals seeking **addiction services**, which are services provided to

* In 2020 The Joint Commission BHC accreditation program announced new and revised child welfare requirements and additional enhancements to standards and EPs to reflect a more humanistic approach to care, treatment, and services. The results were nearly 90 new or revised requirements and updates in language to help organizations create policies and practices that facilitate better outcomes for the children, youth, and families they serve. The changes reflect standards that are culturally sensitive, grounded in trauma-informed care, and more appropriate to a broader range of programs and services.

individuals with substance use disorders or addictive behaviors; for **intensive outpatient programs (IOPs)**; and case planning for **child welfare agencies**. These programs are some of the most common that The Joint Commission accredits. However, it is beyond the scope of this book to address treatment plans for all programs, services, and special populations that The Joint Commission surveys and accredits. To identify requirements applicable to your organization, check the "Standards Applicability Process" (SAP) chapter in the most current version of your *CAMBHC* or its E-dition® counterpart, which includes an applicability grid.

Treatment Plans for Intensive Outpatient Programs

In recent years, the number of individuals with addiction or substance use disorders as well as drug overdoses has risen, due in part to pressures exacerbated by the COVID-19 pandemic. Data from a national study conducted by The Recovery Village in November 2020 revealed that 36% of survey respondents reported an increase in illicit drug use, while 67% of respondents who live in states hardest hit by the pandemic (New York, New Jersey, Massachusetts, Rhode Island, Connecticut) reported an increase in alcohol consumption.[1] In addition, according to estimates released by the US Centers for Disease Control and Prevention, there was a record 100,306 fatal drug overdoses in the United States for the 12 months ending in April 2021. This marks a 28.5% increase from the 12-month period ending April 2020.[2]

IOPs are short-term, acute treatment programs used to address addictions, depression, eating disorders, or other dependencies that do not require detoxification or around-the-clock supervision of the individual served. Substance use recovery and behavioral health care support services provided by IOPs, also known as intensive outpatient treatment (IOT) programs, require unique systemic protocols that blend evidence-based guidelines with cognitive behavioral interventions, relapse prevention training, motivational enhancement, and individualized case management.[3]

To address an increasing need for safe, high-quality care of individuals receiving addiction services, in 2020 The Joint Commission modified requirements in its CTS and "Leadership" (LD) chapters of the *CAMBHC*. The changes were made, in part, to enhance addiction treatment; specifically, providing the appropriate level of care, proper use of drug testing, and transitions of care and follow-up. Here are some of the unique characteristics and common challenges for IOPs related to treatment planning.

Screening Considerations for Individuals with Addiction

Screening and treatment planning requirements for IOPs are not different from those discussed earlier in this book, but it is critical in this setting to capture information that helps determine the level of care needed for the individual served. Based on their screening, individuals seeking treatment for addiction or substance use disorder should be matched to the best level of care, appropriate treatment modalities, and a setting that supports recovery. Inadequate screening and assessment of individuals with substance use disorders may result in care that is inappropriate for the individual's clinical needs, which leads to poor outcomes. It can also mean that the organization is misallocating its resources.

Joint Commission surveyors closely evaluate a facility's screening and assessment processes related to the IOP's entry criteria and how an individual's level of care is determined. At a minimum, a facility's screening processes should capture the common standard screening needs, plus any additional critical information about the individual's medical history, substance use history, and readiness to change, to determine the appropriate level of care.

Screening should include the individual's presenting problems, treatment goals, and recovery needs as well as his or her history of addictive behaviors. Organizations should consider and document during treatment planning whether individuals acquired the substance(s) from a prescription written for them by a medical provider or whether it was acquired in other ways, such as from friends, stolen, or bought off-market.

Because an individual's readiness to change can influence treatment outcomes, the organization must gather such information and factor it into the individual's treatment plan. For example, an individual who is legally mandated for treatment may be unwilling to admit there is a problem, which might indicate that individual is not ready to change. Motivational interviewing, discussed in Chapter 2, can help determine and categorize an individual's level of motivation and provides ways to increase motivation to change. Treatment plans should also account for an individual's recovery/living environment, to ensure that it is supportive, stable, and safe, which has been shown to improve treatment outcomes.

When evaluating an individual's medical and/or recovery history, treatment plans should account for the individual's past and current withdrawal responses and risks for withdrawal symptoms, such as seizures. Assessing withdrawal potential can decrease the likelihood that an individual will return for detoxification treatment and is critical to providing safe, high-quality care.

In many cases, individuals are referred to an IOP as a step-down service from an inpatient or residential setting, or as a step-up from individual or group outpatient treatment. Although individuals may be referred to IOPs, IOPs are required to do their own diligence in terms of screening and assessment and should initiate a new plan of care. Thorough screening and assessment processes will help the organization verify the level of care appropriate for the individual for the best possible care outcome.

Assessment Considerations for Individuals with Addiction

The American Society of Addiction Medicine (ASAM) offers a commonly used set of practice guidelines that meets Joint Commission requirements for a **multidimensional assessment** for addiction,[4] as required in standard CTS.02.03.13, EP 1. The ASAM Criteria, formerly known as the ASAM Patient Placement Criteria, is a comprehensive set of guidelines for determining placement and level of care, continued stay, and transfer and/or discharge of individuals in treatment for addiction and co-occurring conditions. The goal of the ASAM Criteria is to provide outcome-oriented and results-based care in the treatment of addiction by using a multidimensional assessment approach for treatment planning across all levels of care.

This multidimensional approach is meant to create an individualized, holistic, biopsychosocial assessment of an individual by considering all the following domains:[4]

- Acute intoxication and/or withdrawal potential, which explores the individual's current and past experience with substance use and withdrawal.
- Biomedical conditions and complications, which assess an individual's health history and current physical health needs, including nutrition.
- Emotional, behavioral, or cognitive conditions and complications that evaluate an individual's mental health history and any current cognitive and mental health issues and needs.
- Readiness to change explores the individual's interest in and motivation for change.
- Relapse, continued use, or continued problem potential, looks at an individual's unique needs that may influence risk for relapse or continued substance use.
- Recovering, or living environment includes assessing the individual's living situation and the people and/or environment that can either support or hinder the individual's recovery.

This strengths-based multidimensional assessment takes into account individuals' needs, obstacles, and liabilities, as well as strengths, assets, resources, and personal support structure, which together are used to determine the appropriate level of care. Levels of care are defined for adults and adolescents. This approach offers the following benefits to providers and clinicians when planning and developing treatment plans:

- Assisting individuals from assessment through treatment
- Assisting individuals to identify and determine goals
- Ranking and rating levels of risk to determine where to focus treatment and services
- Determining intensity and frequency of interventions using levels of care guidelines

Building Individualized Treatment Plans for Individuals with Addiction

An individualized treatment plan for IOP settings must be developed with input from the individual served to address and identify all areas of need related to the addiction as well as any co-occurring physical, emotional, or mental health disorder(s). IOPs provide a minimum of nine hours of service per week for adults or six hours per week for adolescents. According to the Substance Abuse and Mental Health Services Administration (SAMHSA), the average length of stay in an IOP, for individuals 18 years and older who complete treatment, is 81 days.[5] Keep this in mind as you work to build individualized treatment plans and develop modalities that meet individuals' goals and ensure measurable outcomes within this time frame.

SAMHSA also recommends that IOPs include the following services:

- Individual counseling: At least once a week to discuss issues that individuals may be reluctant to discuss in a group setting.
- Case management: Based on your IOP policies, **case management, or coordination** may include developing the individualized plan, coordinating access to medical or behavioral health services, monitoring program follow-through and outcomes, and advocating for clients who need housing, financial assistance, or vocational services.
- Group counseling and activities: Typically used as the primary treatment modality, group sessions are counselor led and focus on building healthy behaviors through psychoeducation, coping strategies, relapse prevention, and peer support.
- 24-hour crisis services: All IOPs should have 24-hour crisis services to provide intervention emergency services outside the program.
- Family services: IOPs should offer services to families of individuals in treatment to promote healthy home environments and reinforce a supportive recovery environment.

Some recommended optional services include medication-assisted treatment or coordinated services such as childcare and transportation, depending on the organization's scope of service. Due to the intensive nature of the IOP setting, plans of care should be developed immediately. Joint Commission Standard CTS.03.01.03, EP 28, requires organizations providing care, treatment, or services for individuals with addictions to develop treatment plans at the time of admission or entry to care, as this has been shown to lead to better outcomes for the individual served.

Common Goals for Treatment

Although individuals' goals for care, treatment, or services vary, some common goals include the following:

- To achieve abstinence
- To learn and adopt new behaviors that support abstinence and a lifestyle without substance abuse
- To participate in a community-based program for long-term support, such as attending regular meetings at Alcoholics Anonymous
- To identify and find solutions to external problems such as housing, employment, or adherence to probation requirements
- To develop a positive support network
- To improve problem-solving skills and coping strategies

Some studies have shown that individuals with three or more co-occurring issues identified in their treatment plan have a higher IOP retention rate.[6] This may suggest that individuals with more challenges have a greater recognition of the need for treatment. It may also suggest that these individuals may receive more attention from counselors during treatment. As such, and whenever possible, interventions designed to help achieve goals, such as group counseling, should ensure that individuals are matched appropriately with treatment, staff, and others based on their goals and recovery progress.

Routine Testing and Monitoring

A standard practice for IOPs is to routinely monitor individuals being treated for substance use disorders by using drug and/or alcohol consumption tests. Joint Commission Standard CTS.02.03.15, EP 1, requires accredited organizations that provide care, treatment, or services for individuals with addictions to have and to follow a written policy on performing drug testing that is appropriate and based on the individual's diagnosis, progress in treatment, history of use, and clinical judgment. Organizations are also required to document the reason for testing, the results, and the actions taken based on those results. To promote safe quality of care, such organizations are also required to provide education and training to staff involved in drug testing, which—at minimum—includes test administration and specimen storage. These requirements highlight the value of drug testing to assist not only in clinical decision making but also as a therapeutic prompt during discussions about substance use. Testing must be done in a manner that reduces stigma and accounts for the dignity and respect of the individual served. The aim is to aid in the individual's recovery process and not to cause additional harm.

Determining the Next Level of Service

Soliciting and capturing feedback at designated intervals (as determined by the organization) during treatment in an IOP improves outcomes by alerting case managers to the need to modify the treatment plan.[7] Close monitoring and documentation of individuals' progress toward achieving their goals are necessary to determine the next level of care for addiction services. In some cases, this may be a 12-step recovery support group (step down a level) or a residential option if the individual's response to the IOP setting did not successfully improve substance use behaviors (step up a level).

The Center for Substance Abuse Treatment (CSAT)—part of SAMSHA—offers best practice guidelines for treatment planning in IOPs and other settings that treat substance use disorders in adults and adolescents. In CSAT's Treatment Improvement Protocols (TIPs),[8] organizations may find resources that provide quick information as demand for treatment for substance use disorders continues to increase across the country.

Case Plans for Child Welfare Agencies

Currently, there are 17 EPs within Standard CTS.03.02.03 that define expectations for how Joint Commission–accredited child welfare agencies should develop and review case plans. Many of these requirements became effective in 2020 to address areas for enhancing care, treatment, and services related to planning, assessment, reunification, trauma-informed care, and case closing. Changes are aimed to help improve child welfare for individuals and families served by the following services:

- Adoption agencies
- Family preservation
- Foster care
- Respite care
- Kinship care
- Child protective services
- Family reunification services (children's residential centers and group homes)

Like a treatment plan, a **case plan** is an individualized plan for provision of care, treatment, or services. In some cases, a county provides a case plan to a contracted child welfare agency; the plan includes the services needed and the frequency with which to provide service. *Case plan* is the term used by child welfare agencies for the record of care for a case, for which case coordination and case management services are provided. Such services may or may not include clinical treatment or services. This is determined by the organization's policy and the scope of service it is able to and contracted to provide.

During screening and assessment activities, the child welfare agency must make an effort to reach family members or people who play a significant role in the life of the individual served to evaluate relationships. In some cases, particularly in situations of abuse or neglect, this may not be appropriate, or it may be impossible to reach family members (for example, a parent or parents are incarcerated). For Joint Commission compliance, however, efforts made to include family should be documented in the case plan. In addition, and as part of assessment activities, the agency must do the following:

- Evaluate barriers to placement along with any concerns from the individual served or the **resource family** (or **resource parent**). Barriers to successful placement include, for example, placement far away from the child's school or community, or a child may have special needs or a medical condition that can make successful placement challenging.
- Evaluate the family's strengths and opportunities for growth.

A Trauma-Informed Case Plan

Chapter 1 defined trauma and addressed strategies for **trauma-informed care**. Joint Commission–compliant case plans for child welfare services should be trauma-informed. To be precise, Standard CTS.02.04.01, EP 18, requires that, as part of routine screening and assessment practices, assessments must be trauma-informed for this setting. Also, as required by Standard CTS.03.02.03, EP 2, the comprehensive assessment must be based on the emotional, behavioral, developmental, educational, spiritual, social, physical, cultural, linguistic, and legal status of the individual served as well as that of the family of origin, such as the individual's caregiver and/or parent.

Trauma-informed case planning begins with screening and assessment activities designed to identify individuals who may have experienced trauma, abuse, neglect, or exploitation. When youth are at risk of neglect, domestic violence, sexual exploitation, elopement, or sexually reactive behaviors, a preliminary plan of care may be necessary to ensure immediate safety (as discussed in Chapter 1). This book has emphasized repeatedly that all treatment plans should be individualized, and when building the case plan for child welfare services, the same is true. Screening and assessments in child welfare cases should include the following:

- Learning about a child's trauma history, identifying current symptoms and functional delays, and identifying children who need additional assessment and possible treatment
- Conducting a detailed clinical evaluation of children whose trauma screen indicates trauma history, combined with psychological symptoms and/or functional delays, as the basis for case planning
- Gathering data about a child's strengths, needs, and preferences, and measuring improvements in skills and competencies to inform ongoing case planning
- Measuring outcomes to ensure that services are achieving desired results at the child's level, and, if not, evaluating, revising, and updating the case plan, as needed

Screening and Assessment Tools for Child Welfare

The Child and Adolescent Needs and Strengths (CANS) is a multipurpose tool developed for children's services and is frequently used for measuring outcomes in child welfare programs to help identify and address the needs of traumatized children and families.[9] Practitioners can use the CANS to support clinical decision making, including level of care and placement decisions; linking the findings of the assessment to individualized service and treatment plans; engaging family members in the assessment process; and facilitating the planning and evaluation of the service provided to drive performance improvement.

Although several versions of the CANS have been developed or adapted for use within particular states or child-serving systems, the standard form (*see* Tool 4-1 on page 75) uses the following domains for assessment:

- **Life functioning**, such as family, social, and living situation
- **Individual strengths**, including optimism, talents and interests, cultural identity, and so on
- **Cultural factors**, such as language, traditions and rituals, and cultural stress
- **Caregiver resources and needs** (for example, available supervision, level of involvement with care, residential stability)
- **Behavioral/emotional needs**, including trauma and substance use disorder, depression, anxiety, oppositional disorder, attachment difficulties, and so on
- **Risk behaviors** (for example, suicide risk, self-harm, danger to others)

Staff Requirements

When developing the trauma-informed case plan, staff should address potential triggering behaviors or conditions (such as the individual's personal space, type of touch preferred, and so on), risk and protective factors, and community resources that are available to alleviate the effects of maltreatment of children and youth and prevent future trauma. In addition, staff should participate in training specific to their job responsibilities, which means that if staff are required to assess trauma in young children, then they must be trained and competent to do so. This is outlined in the "Human Resources Management" (HRM) chapter under Standard HRM.01.05.01. All child welfare agency staff should demonstrate cultural and age-specific competence (*see* HRM.01.06.01, EP 7).

It is important to note that effective training for a trauma-informed practice requires comprehensive training that cannot be accomplished in a single workshop. Trauma-informed training may be more effective if child welfare staff are cross-trained with professionals from partner agencies and systems, so that all child-serving systems can work together in the best interests of children and families served. The Joint Commission requires child welfare agencies to determine appropriate training and establish a process to evaluate staff for competency.

The Permanency Goal

The case plan should identify the permanency goal, resolution, or a long-term solution to establish long-term bonds and promote stability, safety, and well-being if the individual is a child or youth in an out-of-home placement or foster care. **Permanency planning** is the process of assisting the transition of children from a biological parent(s) to a foster home or other care provider for the purpose of providing a child with a safe, stable, environment. Federal law requires states to establish a permanency plan for children in foster care (that is, a plan for where children will live when they leave foster care—whether they go home to family [reunification], live permanently with a relative [kinship care], or are placed for adoption), or are released from the custody/control of parents or guardian and allowed to exercise control over their own lives [emancipation]. Often, emancipation occurs by law at age 18, but this may vary by state and other considerations.)

Permanency planning requires Joint Commission–accredited agencies to consider input from all parties involved and is reviewed according to law and regulation. For example, when the permanency goal is placement in a living arrangement outside the family home, some state laws require that the child welfare agency document reasons it is not in the child's best interest to return to the family home because the local court system will make its final determination based on those factors.

Assessing for Permanency

An agency's case plan should document assessment for potential reunification or other potential permanency options. If reunification with family is possible and appropriate, then it is the preferred goal, but if reunification is not appropriate, then adoption is often considered to provide the greatest degree of permanence. However, in some situations, adoption may not be an appropriate option, such as with older children who may object to losing legal ties to their birth parents or for children with special needs that might limit options for placement in a home environment. In such cases, the permanency option may be guardianship with relatives. Although permanency options and requirements vary by state, many statutes addressing legal permanency options include the following[10]:

- Reunification with parents
- Adoption, with placement preference given to a relative or current foster parent
- Permanent placement and legal guardianship with a fit and willing relative (kinship care)
- Legal guardianship or custody with another adult who is not a relative
- Another planned permanent living arrangement, such as long-term foster care, residential care, or independent living.*

The case plan should also include, at a minimum, short- and long-term goals (successful visitation or reunification), arrangements of services (such as facilitating necessary medical appointments, sources of support (such as therapist), how the agency will help the family transition, and how it will advocate on the family's behalf, such as in cases that require court determinations.

Although the overarching goal is to meet the child's needs, a Joint Commission–compliant case plan must also address goals the family is expected to meet in a desired time frame, and how the agency will help the family meet those goals. For example, a court may determine that the child's mother must complete a substance use counseling program before the child is allowed to return home. The child welfare agency can assist the family by referring the mother to an appropriate provider and discuss her progress during family meetings to encourage her to achieve that goal.

Finally, the case planning process should assess preparation for transitional living when older youth or adults are discharged from foster care. Services and activities that can help these individuals develop skills necessary for independence include the following:

- Employment career planning assessments
- Financial management
- Daily living skills (for example, cooking, transportation)
- Completing high school, general educational development (GED), or college
- Job search training
- Vocational training
- Parenting skills
- Developing social/relationship skills and support systems

* In 38 states (as of February 2020), when the permanency goal is another planned permanent living arrangement (APPLA), the child welfare agency must document compelling reasons why other permanency options are not in the child's best interest, and in 24 states, the child must be at least 16 years old before APPLA may be selected as the permanency goal (US Department of Health and Human Services, Children's Bureau, Child Welfare Information Gateway. Court Hearings for the Permanent Placement of Children. 2020. Accessed Dec 24, 2021. https://www.childwelfare.gov/pubPDFs/planning.pdf.

After-Care Planning

After-care planning requires agency follow-up, as appropriate, or referral of an individual to an appropriate agency. An after-care plan should consider the needs of different types of adoptive families, such as relatives, or foster families who adopt, or families that only foster. The Joint Commission requires the agency to provide resources that identify support systems for youth as they transition to adulthood. For individuals who age out of the foster care system, this may include access to specific activities offered by the child welfare agency, or to other community agencies that can provide tutoring, parenting classes, job and career skills training, or temporary financial assistance, for example.

An unfortunate side effect for many children in family displacement situations is acute mental health disorder. If necessary, agencies accredited by The Joint Commission are to refer children to appropriate mental health services when the need is identified and the care required is outside the agency's scope of service.

Like treatment plans, case plans should be periodically reviewed, evaluated, and revised according to the organization's policy but also with considerations for relevant state laws and federal regulations. Evaluations may include agency staff, cross-sector contacts, the individual served, the foster parent(s), the family of origin (for children and youth only), or a representative of the state authority. Case plan review is required to accurately track an individual's progress and to help the family continue to meet its goals.

Summary

This chapter focuses on a few unique examples of populations served and services offered by BHC organizations, but there are many others. The goal here is to build on the common standards that apply to all organizations accredited under the BHC program umbrellas and also address additional treatment planning requirements for individuals seeking complex care, treatment, or services. In the next chapter, we will explore a few typical case scenarios and offer sample treatment plans for the individuals profiled in the sample scenarios.

References

1. The Recovery Village. Drug and Alcohol Use Increase During COVID-19. LaNeve N, editor. (Updated: Dec 17, 2020.) Accessed Dec 24, 2021. https://www.therecoveryvillage.com/drug-addiction/news/drug-alcohol-use-rising-during-covid/.

2. Everyday Health. U.S. Drug Overdose Deaths Continue to Surge During COVID-19 Pandemic. Rapaport L. Nov 24, 2021. Accessed Dec 24, 2021. https://www.everydayhealth.com/opioid-addiction/us-drug-overdose-deaths-continue-to-surge-during-covid-19-pandemic/.

3. Substance Abuse and Mental Health Services Administration, Center for Substance Abuse Treatment. Substance Abuse: *Clinical Issues in Intensive Outpatient Treatment*. Treatment Improvement Protocol (TIP) 47. DHHS Publication No. (SMA) 06-4182. 2006. Accessed Dec 24, 2021. https://store.samhsa.gov/sites/default/files/d7/priv/sma13-4182.pdf.

4. American Society of Addiction Medicine. The ASAM Criteria. Accessed Dec 24, 2021. https://www.asam.org/asam-criteria.

5. Substance Abuse and Mental Health Services Administration. *Advisory: Clinical Issues in Intensive Outpatient Treatment for Substance Use Disorders*. Publication No. PEP20-02-01-021. 2021. Accessed Dec 24, 2021. https://store.samhsa.gov/sites/default/files/SAMHSA_Digital_Download/pep20-02-01-021.pdf.

6. Veach LJ, et al. Retention predictors related to intensive outpatient programs for substance use disorders. *Am J Drug Alcohol Abuse*. 2009 Aug;26(3):417–428.

7. Kuusisto K, Lintonen T. Factors predicting satisfaction in outpatient substance abuse treatment: A prospective follow-up study. *Subst Abuse Treat Prev Policy*. 2020 May 24;15(1):35.

8. Substance Abuse and Mental Health Services Administration. SAMHSA/CSAT Treatment Improvement Protocols. 1993–. Accessed Dec 24, 2021. https://www.ncbi.nlm.nih.gov/books/NBK82999/.

9. Praed Foundation. The Child and Adolescent Needs and Strengths (CANS). Accessed Dec 24, 2021. https://praedfoundation.org/tcom/tcom-tools/the-child-and-adolescent-needs-and-strengths-cans/.

10. US Department of Health and Human Services, Children's Bureau, Child Welfare Information Gateway. Court Hearings for the Permanent Placement of Children. 2020. Accessed Dec 24, 2021. https://www.childwelfare.gov/topics/systemwide/laws-policies/statutes/planning/.

Tool 4-1. Standard Comprehensive Child and Adolescent Needs and Strengths (CANS) 3.0 Rating Sheet

DOWNLOAD

Date:			
Type: ☐ Initial ☐ Scheduled Update ☐ Major Life Event ☐ Exit			
Assessor ID:		Program:	
Client Name:		Client ID:	DOB
Gender:	Ethnicity:	Grade:	Zip Code:

For the **Life Functioning Domain and associated module**, use the following categories and action levels:

0 – No current need; no need for action or intervention.

1 – Identified need that requires monitoring, watchful waiting, or preventive action based on history, suspicion, or disagreement.

2 – Action is required to ensure that the identified need is addressed; need is interfering with functioning.

3 – Need is dangerous or disabling; requires immediate and/or intensive action.

LIFE FUNCTIONING DOMAIN

Items	N/A	0	1	2	3		0	1	2	3
Family Functioning		☐	☐	☐	☐	Medical/Physical	☐	☐	☐	☐
Living Situation		☐	☐	☐	☐	Sexual Development	☐	☐	☐	☐
Social Functioning		☐	☐	☐	☐	Sleep	☐	☐	☐	☐
Recreational		☐	☐	☐	☐	School Attendance	☐	☐	☐	☐
Developmental/Intellectual (A)		☐	☐	☐	☐	School Behavior	☐	☐	☐	☐
Job Functioning	☐	☐	☐	☐	☐	School Achievement	☐	☐	☐	☐
Legal		☐	☐	☐	☐	Decision Making	☐	☐	☐	☐
A. DEVELOPMENTAL NEEDS MODULE *(To complete when the Developmental/Intellectual item is rated "1," "2," or "3.")*										
Cognitive		☐	☐	☐	☐	*Communication*	☐	☐	☐	☐
Developmental		☐	☐	☐	☐	*Self-Care/ Daily Living Skills*	☐	☐	☐	☐

Please write a rationale for any item in the above domain or modules rated actionable ("2" or "3").

Page **1** of **7**

For the **Individual Strengths**, use the following categories and action levels:

0 – Well-developed centerpiece strength; may be used as a centerpiece in an intervention/action plan.

1 – Identified and useful strength. Strength will be used, maintained, or built upon as part of the plan. May require some effort to develop strength into a centerpiece strength.

2 – Strengths have been identified but require strength-building efforts before they can be effectively utilized as part of a plan. Identified but not useful.

3 – An area in which no current strength is identified; efforts may be recommended to develop a strength in this area.

INDIVIDUAL STRENGTHS DOMAIN

Items	N/A	0	1	2	3		0	1	2	3
Family Strengths		☐	☐	☐	☐	Community Life	☐	☐	☐	☐
Interpersonal		☐	☐	☐	☐	Relationship Permanence	☐	☐	☐	☐
Optimism		☐	☐	☐	☐	Resilience	☐	☐	☐	☐
Educational Setting	☐	☐	☐	☐	☐	Resourcefulness	☐	☐	☐	☐
Vocational		☐	☐	☐	☐	Cultural Identity	☐	☐	☐	☐
Talents and Interests		☐	☐	☐	☐	Natural Supports	☐	☐	☐	☐
Spiritual/Religious		☐	☐	☐	☐		☐	☐	☐	☐

Please write a rationale for Centerpiece ("0") and Useful ("1") Strengths, as well as Strengths to Build ("2" or "3").

Page **2** of **7**

For the **Cultural Factors Domain**, use the following categories and action levels:

0 – No current need; no need for action or intervention.

1 – Identified need that requires monitoring, watchful waiting, or preventive action based on history, suspicion, or disagreement.

2 – Action is required to ensure that the identified need is addressed; need is interfering with functioning.

3 – Need is dangerous or disabling; requires immediate and/or intensive action.

CULTURAL FACTORS DOMAIN

Items	0	1	2	3		0	1	2	3
Language	☐	☐	☐	☐	Cultural Stress	☐	☐	☐	☐
Traditions and Rituals	☐	☐	☐	☐					

Please write a rationale for any item in the above domain rated actionable ("2" or "3").

CAREGIVER RESOURCES & NEEDS DOMAIN ☐ Not applicable; no caregiver identified.

0 – No current need; no need for action or intervention. This may be a resource for the child/youth.

1 – Identified need that requires monitoring, watchful waiting, or preventive action based on history, suspicion, or disagreement. This may be an opportunity for resource building.

2 – Need is interfering with the provision of care; action is required to ensure that the identified need is addressed.

3 – Need prevents the provision of care; requires immediate and/or intensive action.

Page **3** of **7**

Items	0	1	2	3		0	1	2	3
Supervision	☐	☐	☐	☐	Medical/Physical	☐	☐	☐	☐
Involvement with Care	☐	☐	☐	☐	Mental Health	☐	☐	☐	☐
Knowledge	☐	☐	☐	☐	Substance Use	☐	☐	☐	☐
Organization	☐	☐	☐	☐	Developmental	☐	☐	☐	☐
Social Resources	☐	☐	☐	☐	Safety	☐	☐	☐	☐
Residential Stability	☐	☐	☐	☐					

Please write a rationale for any item in the domain above rated actionable ("2" or "3").

For the **Behavioral/Emotional Needs Domain and associated modules**, use the following categories and action levels:

0 – No current need; no need for action or intervention.

1 – Identified need that requires monitoring, watchful waiting, or preventive action based on history, suspicion, or disagreement.

2 – Action is required to ensure that the identified need is addressed; need is interfering with functioning.

3 – Need is dangerous or disabling; requires immediate and/or intensive action.

BEHAVIORAL/EMOTIONAL NEEDS DOMAIN

Items	0	1	2	3		0	1	2	3
Psychosis (Thought Disorder)	☐	☐	☐	☐	Conduct (Antisocial Behavior)	☐	☐	☐	☐
Impulsivity/Hyperactivity	☐	☐	☐	☐	*Adjustment to Trauma (B)*	☐	☐	☐	☐
Depression	☐	☐	☐	☐	Attachment Difficulties	☐	☐	☐	☐
Anxiety	☐	☐	☐	☐	Anger Control	☐	☐	☐	☐
Oppositional	☐	☐	☐	☐	*Substance Use (C)*	☐	☐	☐	☐

Page **4** of **7**

B. TRAUMA MODULE *(To complete when the Adjustment to Trauma item is rated "1," "2," or "3.")*

For the **Traumatic/Adverse Childhood Experiences**, use the following categories and action levels:

No – No evidence of any trauma of this type.

Yes – Child/youth has had experience, or there is suspicion that the child/youth has experienced this type of trauma—one incident, multiple incidents, or chronic, on-going experiences.

B1. Traumatic/Adverse Childhood Exp.	**No**	**Yes**		**No**	**Yes**
Sexual Abuse	☐	☐	*Witness to Family Violence*	☐	☐
Physical Abuse	☐	☐	*Witness to Comm./School Violence*	☐	☐
Neglect	☐	☐	*War/Terrorism Affected*	☐	☐
Emotional Abuse	☐	☐	*Witness /Victim of Criminal Acts*	☐	☐
Medical Trauma	☐	☐	*Parental Criminal Behavior*	☐	☐
Natural or Man-Made Disaster	☐	☐	*Disrupt in Caregiving/Attchmt Losses*	☐	☐
Sexual Abuse	☐	☐	*Witness to Family Violence*	☐	☐

Items	**0**	**1**	**2**	**3**		**0**	**1**	**2**	**3**
B2. Traumatic Stress Symptoms									
Emotional and/or Phys. Dysregulation	☐	☐	☐	☐	*Avoidance*	☐	☐	☐	☐
Intrusions / Reexperiencing	☐	☐	☐	☐	*Numbing*	☐	☐	☐	☐
Traumatic Grief	☐	☐	☐	☐	*Dissociation*	☐	☐	☐	☐
Hyperarousal	☐	☐	☐	☐	*Time Before Treatment*	☐	☐	☐	☐
C. SUBSTANCE USE DISORDER MODULE *(To complete when the Substance Use item is rated "1," "2," or "3.")*									
Severity of Use	☐	☐	☐	☐	*Parental Influences*	☐	☐	☐	☐
Duration of Use	☐	☐	☐	☐	*Environmental Influences*	☐	☐	☐	☐
Stage of Recovery	☐	☐	☐	☐	*Recovery Support in Community*	☐	☐	☐	☐
Peer Influences	☐	☐	☐	☐					

Please write a rationale for any item in the above domain or module rated actionable ("2" or "3").

Page **5** of **7**

For the **Risk Behaviors Domain and associated modules**, use the following categories and action levels:

0 – No current need; no need for action or intervention.

1 – Identified need that requires monitoring, watchful waiting, or preventive action based on history, suspicion, or disagreement.

2 – Action is required to ensure that the identified need is addressed; need is interfering with functioning.

3 – Need is dangerous or disabling; requires immediate and/or intensive action.

RISK BEHAVIORS DOMAIN

Items	0	1	2	3		0	1	2	3
Suicide Risk	☐	☐	☐	☐	*Runaway (F)*	☐	☐	☐	☐
Non-Suicidal Self-Injurious Behavior	☐	☐	☐	☐	*Delinquent Behavior (G)*	☐	☐	☐	☐
Other Self-Harm (Recklessness)	☐	☐	☐	☐	*Fire Setting (H)*	☐	☐	☐	☐
Danger to Others (D)	☐	☐	☐	☐	Intentional Misbehavior	☐	☐	☐	☐
Sexual Aggression (E)	☐	☐	☐	☐					
D. DANGEROUSNESS/VIOLENCE MODULE *(To complete when the Danger to Others item is rated "1," "2," or "3.")*									
History of Violence	☐	☐	☐	☐	*Violent Thinking*	☐	☐	☐	☐
Frustration Management	☐	☐	☐	☐	*Aware of Violence Potential*	☐	☐	☐	☐
Hostility	☐	☐	☐	☐	*Response to Consequences*	☐	☐	☐	☐
Paranoid Thinking	☐	☐	☐	☐	*Commitment to Self-Control*	☐	☐	☐	☐
Secondary Gains from Anger	☐	☐	☐	☐	*Treatment Involvement*	☐	☐	☐	☐
E. SEXUALLY AGGRESSIVE BEHAVIOR MODULE *(To complete when the Sexual Aggression item is rated "1," "2," or "3.")*									
Relationship	☐	☐	☐	☐	*Type of Sex Act*	☐	☐	☐	☐
Physical Force/Threat	☐	☐	☐	☐	*Response to Accusation*	☐	☐	☐	☐
Planning	☐	☐	☐	☐	*Temporal Consistency*	☐	☐	☐	☐

Page **6** of **7**

Age Differential	☐	☐	☐	☐	*History of Sexually Aggressive Behav.*	☐	☐	☐	☐
F. RUNAWAY MODULE *(To complete when the Runaway item is rated "1," "2," or "3.")*									
Frequency of Running	☐	☐	☐	☐	*Likelihood of Return on Own*	☐	☐	☐	☐
Consistency of Destination	☐	☐	☐	☐	*Involvement with Others*	☐	☐	☐	☐
Safety of Destination	☐	☐	☐	☐	*Realistic Expectations*	☐	☐	☐	☐
Involvement in Illegal Activities	☐	☐	☐	☐	*Planning*	☐	☐	☐	☐

Items	0	1	2	3		0	1	2	3
G. JUVENILE JUSTICE MODULE *(To complete when the Delinquent Behavior item is rated "1," "2," or "3.")*									
History	☐	☐	☐	☐	*Peer Influences*	☐	☐	☐	☐
Seriousness	☐	☐	☐	☐	*Parental Criminal Behavior*	☐	☐	☐	☐
Planning	☐	☐	☐	☐	*Environmental Influences*	☐	☐	☐	☐
Community Safety	☐	☐	☐	☐	*Legal Compliance*	☐	☐	☐	☐
H. FIRE SETTING MODULE *(To complete when the Fire Setting item is rated "1," "2," or "3.")*									
History	☐	☐	☐	☐	*Community Safety*	☐	☐	☐	☐
Seriousness	☐	☐	☐	☐	*Response to Accusation*	☐	☐	☐	☐
Planning	☐	☐	☐	☐	*Remorse*	☐	☐	☐	☐
Use of Accelerants	☐	☐	☐	☐	*Likelihood of Future Fire Setting*	☐	☐	☐	☐
Intention to Harm	☐	☐	☐	☐					

Please write a rationale for any item in the above domain or modules rated actionable ("2" or "3").

Source: John Praed Foundation. Dec 2020. Accessed Dec 24, 2021. https://praedfoundation.org/tcom/tcom-tools/the-child-and-adolescent-needs-and-strengths-cans/.

Page **7** of **7**

Chapter 5
Sample Cases and Treatment Plans

The following case scenarios are examples of typical encounters for organizations that offer behavioral health care, treatment, and services. These scenarios and corresponding sample treatment plans are meant to provide examples and context to demonstrate how treatment planning and execution processes might play out for an individual served.

Case #1: Ralph J.

Ralph J. is a 40-year-old man who visited an outpatient behavioral health facility upon referral from his company's employee assistance program. Ralph works as an air traffic controller, a job he has held for 15 years. His work performance has deteriorated recently following the sudden and unexpected death of his older brother—with whom he was very close—from a heart attack at age 44. Ralph has had difficulty concentrating and sleeping. He is mourning his brother and obsessed with worry that the same thing might happen to him. He has a sedentary lifestyle, is 40 pounds overweight, and has smoked since age 17. At his last physical three years ago, his physician indicated Ralph was prediabetic, but he has avoided seeing his physician because he has made no changes to his diet or activity level.

Ralph is married with a son and a daughter who are currently a senior and a junior in high school, respectively. Ralph's wife, who works part-time in a retail job during school hours, is frustrated with Ralph's inability to get beyond his brother's death and upset that he recently received a disciplinary action at work for excessive tardiness and falling asleep on the job. Ralph and his wife have been arguing frequently. Ralph is the primary wage earner, and the family relies on his employment benefits. The family is counting on his income to pay the children's upcoming college tuition. Ralph is reluctant to engage in treatment because he feels a man should be able to handle this on his own and is afraid of his coworkers' reactions if they find out he is seeking behavioral health care.

Two months after beginning treatment, Ralph is laid off from work due to the COVID-19 pandemic–related decrease in travel, and he becomes increasingly depressed and panicked about how he will support his family. He feels he has become a burden and begins to wonder if they would be better off without him. The first anniversary of his brother's death is approaching, and Ralph fantasizes about visiting his brother's grave and shooting himself with the deer rifle he has from when he and his brother used to go hunting together.

Sample Treatment Plan for Ralph J.

Presenting issues/identified needs: difficulty concentrating, difficulty sleeping, anxiety/depressive symptoms, grief/loss

At admission: Patient Health Questionnaire-9 (PHQ-9) score of 13, indicating moderate depression

Release to wife obtained, invited to attend initial session to review the plan with Ralph's consent.

Long-Term Goal:
Ralph states that he wants "to feel like my old self again and get my health on track. He describes this as being able to focus more during the day, sleep consistently at night, and feel less anxious.

Goals

Goal 1: Increase focus and concentration and reduce feelings of anxiety evidenced by a lowering of PHQ-9 score.

Active/Completed/Referred/Deferred:

Objective 1.1:
Identify negative self-talk messages that contribute to Ralph's anxiety and depression and replace them with positive self-talk.

Intervention 1.1:
Cognitive behavioral therapy during once-a-week individual therapy

Objective 1.2:
Develop and implement mindfulness practices to reduce anxiety and increase focus.

Intervention 1.2:
Cognitive behavioral therapy and mindfulness training during once-a-week individual therapy

Goal 2: Progress through the grief process regarding the loss of Ralph's brother.

Active/Completed/Referred/Deferred:

Objective 2.1:
Identify the stages of grief and Ralph's status in the grief process.

Intervention 2.1:
Individual therapy once a week, focusing on grief work

Objective 2.2:
Develop ways to facilitate movement through the grief process.

Intervention 2.2:
Individual therapy once a week, focusing on grief work

Goal 3: Engage with primary care physician to assess sleep difficulties and develop prediabetes care plan.

Active/Completed/**Referred**/Deferred:
Referral made ________ [date]. Release of Information signed. Letter sent requesting coordination.

Objective 3.1:
Determine health impact on sleep difficulties and initiate prediabetes care plan.

Intervention 3.1:
Ralph to schedule with primary care physician; clinician to coordinate care with primary care physician.

Goal 4: Identify motivation for smoking cessation.

Active/Completed/Referred/**Deferred:** Will be revisited after Ralph has engaged with his physician to address prediabetes.

Review of plan monthly

Month 1:

Goal 1: Increase focus and concentration and reduce feelings of anxiety evidenced by a lowering of PHQ-9 score.

Active/Completed/Referred/Deferred:

Review of progress: Ralph has experienced improvement in depressive symptoms, as evidenced by a reduction in PHQ-9 score from 13 to a score of 11 at this review. He has identified two negative self-talk messages and has become proficient in replacing one with positive self-talk and is currently working on the second. He has recently implemented daily relaxation breathing at lunchtime to work on mindfulness.

Goal 2: Progress through the grief process regarding the loss of Ralph's brother.

Active/Completed/Referred/Deferred:

Review of progress: Ralph has identified that he is currently in the depression stage of grief and is exploring options for celebrating his brother's life that he feels would be meaningful to him.

Goal 3: Engage with primary care physician to assess sleep difficulties and develop prediabetes care plan.

Active/Completed/**Referred**/Deferred:
Referral made ________ [date]. Release of Information signed. Letter sent requesting coordination.

Review of progress: Ralph has scheduled an appointment to meet with his primary care physician for ________ [date].

Goal 4: Identify motivation for smoking cessation.

Active/Completed/Referred/**Deferred**: Will be revisited after Ralph has engaged with his physician to address prediabetes.

Month 2:

Goal 1: Increase focus and concentration and reduce feelings of anxiety evidenced by a lowering of PHQ-9 score.

Active/Completed/Referred/Deferred:

Objective 1.1:
Identify negative self-talk messages that contribute to Ralph's anxiety and depression and replace them with positive self-talk.

Intervention 1.1:
Increased cognitive behavioral therapy to during twice-weekly individual therapy.

Objective 1.2:
Develop and implement mindfulness practices to reduce anxiety and increase focus.

Intervention 1.2:
Increased cognitive behavioral therapy and mindfulness training to during twice-weekly individual therapy.

Review of progress: PHQ-9 score this review increased to 17 from last score of 11 and noted several days Ralph thought he would be better off dead, prompting a suicide risk assessment. Depressive symptoms increasing due to job layoff. Service frequency increased to twice a week, and goal added to address suicide risk: see Goal 5.

Goal 2: Progress through the grief process regarding the loss of Ralph's brother.

Active/Completed/Referred/**Deferred:** This will be deferred until after stabilization from suicidal ideation and current job crisis.
Review of progress: Prior to his job layoff, Ralph had identified a celebratory activity he wanted to implement to honor his brother. This will be deferred until after stabilization from suicidal ideation and current job crisis.

Goal 3: Engage with primary care physician to assess sleep difficulties and develop prediabetes care plan.

Active/Completed/**Referred**/Deferred: Referral made ________ [date]. Release of Information signed. Letter sent requesting coordination.

Objective 3.1:
Determine health impact on sleep difficulties, and initiate prediabetes care plan.

Intervention 3.1:
Ralph to schedule with primary care physician; clinician to coordinate care with primary care physician.

Review of progress: Ralph met with his primary care physician and discussed a plan for his diet and exercise. His primary care physician also made a referral to Sleep Medicine to be considered for an evaluation for a sleep study.

Goal 4: Identify motivation for smoking cessation.

Active/Completed/Referred/**Deferred:** Will be revisited after Ralph has engaged with his physician to address prediabetes.

Goal 5: Create a plan for safety to address suicidal ideation.

Active/Completed/Referred/Deferred:

Objective 5.1:

Complete safety plan and have rifle removed from the home.

Intervention 5.1:

Couple session with Ralph and his wife to review safety plan and confirm rifle has been removed from the home.

Goal 6: Secure new employment.

Active/Completed/**Referred**/Deferred: Referred Ralph to Employment Commission and multiple employment agencies for job search assistance.

Case #2: Sheryl B.

Sheryl B. is a 57-year-old, twice-divorced woman who has been adjudicated to treatment for substance abuse following a car accident. She was speeding, sideswiped another vehicle, and ran off the road. Her blood alcohol level was 0.23 at the time of the crash. At her court hearing, the judge remanded Sheryl to an addiction treatment program.

Sheryl readily admits to regular drinking to cope with feelings of anxiety, but states that she normally limits herself to two drinks per night and that it helps keep her on an even keel. The night of the accident, she was with a group celebrating a friend's upcoming divorce and says she "might have" had three or four drinks. During discussions with Sheryl, she reveals that she grew up in an alcoholic family. Both parents drank, her father regularly and to excess, and her mother less so but to keep him company and "maintain the peace" in the family. She divulges that her father could become combative and abusive when drinking—both verbally and physically. She tried to stay away from these situations but says both she and her two brothers sometimes were the focus of her father's anger, particularly as they grew into adolescence. Sheryl describes her father's behavior as "unpredictable" and her mother as "powerless to intervene in his rages." He was particularly enraged when Sheryl began dating and frequently called her a "slut" and accused her of sleeping with any boy she went out with. On multiple occasions, her father slapped her.

Sheryl left high school at 16 to get away from her family and went to work in a factory. After two months, she married a man twice her age whom she met at a local bar. She says their social life centered around meeting friends at the bar and that drinking was not a problem for her. Occasionally, she also used marijuana and, on a few occasions, cocaine. She became pregnant after her marriage but miscarried at four months. After 15 years of marriage with no further pregnancies, her husband became disabled after a work injury and began drinking heavily. He blamed his drinking on not being able to work and on his disappointment with her for not being able to get pregnant. They eventually divorced.

Following the divorce, Sheryl got her general equivalency diploma (GED) and a new job and is currently an assistant manager at an insurance company. She remarried within a year to a man she met through work, and they adopted a son who is now 23 and in graduate school across the country. She and her second husband drank regularly, but she says not to excess. He was a salesman who traveled frequently for work, and she drank more during his absence to combat her loneliness. They drifted apart as his career progressed, and he initiated a divorce a year ago to marry a younger professional colleague.

Two things have happened in the past month that Sheryl says have been "devastating." Her ex-husband's new wife is now pregnant. She began drinking much more heavily and had a falling-out with her son when he visited during the holidays. He told her that her behavior was out of control, and he was embarrassed by her. He recently became engaged and has not introduced her to his fiancée. She fears her son is cutting her out of his life. Sheryl always wanted a large family and, not having that, has invested all her emotional energy in her son. She feels she has been a failure as a mother and a wife.

Sample Treatment Plan for Sheryl B.

Presenting issues/identified needs: Fulfilling court order, anxiety, trauma history, fear of estrangement from son, grief/loss

Sheryl refused contact with son or other family for involvement in treatment.

Client-stated goal

"I want to get out from under this charge and get back to my life."

Goal 1: Complete recommended substance use disorder treatment.

Active/Completed/Referred/Deferred:

Objective 1.1

Identify influence of substance use on functioning and determine healthier coping strategies to implement.

Intervention 1.1

Substance use outpatient individual and group therapy weekly. Individual therapy once a week and group therapy once a week.

Goal 2: Address history of trauma.

Active/Completed/Referred/**Deferred**: Sheryl has been identified has having experienced past abuse; however, she declined addressing these issues. She was given a list of trauma therapy specialists in the area to access to address this history. This will be deferred as she works on her substance use goal.

Developing the Written Treatment Plan

The sample treatment plans in this chapter offer examples of key points to consider when presented with an individual seeking care. When preparing individualized treatment plans it is important to include the following elements:

- The individual's personal information, psychological history, and demographics
- Diagnoses (diagnostic summary, or summary statement) of the individual's behavioral health issues
- Short-term and long-term goals and expected outcomes
- Measurable objectives
- Interventions and/or treatment modalities
- Timeline for review of treatment progress

Tool 5-1 on page 91 is a development template that includes key points to consider when developing written treatment plans. The template can be adapted to capture all the information that should be included in treatment plans based on organization policies to help ensure documentation of all required information on the individual as well as what is required by laws and federal regulations.

Evaluating the Treatment Plan for Improvement

One way to improve compliance with Joint Commission requirements for treatment planning is to evaluate all planning activities, policies, and procedures; care plans; and records of care on a regular basis. This can be done using the following activities:

- Create a checklist for staff with the key elements of performance (EPs) that may require clarification.
- Compare a sampling of treatment plans against accreditation requirements for a particular setting, service, or individual to identify compliant and noncompliant areas, and then focus on activities, such as tracer activities, to improve areas of noncompliance.
- Use tracer activities to determine how data are used to monitor and inform progress, including records review, conversations with individuals, clinicians, treatment teams, and team supervisors.

An individualized plan of care will include a variety of clinical/case records, such as screening and assessment data, progress notes, and other required documentation. "Record of Care, Treatment, and Services" (RC) Standard RC.01.04.01 requires that behavioral health care and human services (BHC) organizations audit their clinical/case records in accordance with a time frame defined in organization policies. This review will help confirm that information is present, accurate, legible, authenticated, and completed in a timely manner.

A treatment plan evaluation checklist that contains criteria common to all BHC programs/settings may be useful when reviewing individualized treatment plans (*see* Tool 5-2 on page 100). In cases in which more specific criteria are required for an organization's scope of service, this tool can be adapted for use.

Summary

This chapter offers two sample scenarios and corresponding treatment plans to help practitioners and treatment planners better understand how to apply Joint Commission requirements for a typical encounter with an individual served. In addition, a template is provided for consideration when developing a written treatment plan, as well as a checklist to help evaluate the quality of your organization's treatment plans. Both can help improve the overall quality of treatment planning in your organization by helping to identify and capture key points to consider when developing new plans and evaluating existing plans for effectiveness.

By taking a deep dive into the processes and activities that make up effective treatment planning, throughout this book, we aim to help BHC organizations identify and improve their practices and also address compliance issues related to planning for care, treatment, or services. We highlight several areas organizations find challenging, such as incorporating the individual's needs, strengths, preferences, and goals identified during screening and assessment into the treatment plan; ensuring that the treatment plan is individualized and that the individual served is actively involved in decision making; and ensuring that the treatment plan is regularly reviewed, revised, and updated as needed and according to the organization's policy.

As a result of the ongoing COVID-19 pandemic—and the loss and uncertainty it brings—millions continue to be affected by behavioral health issues, which means the demand for behavioral health care has never been higher. BHC organizations are increasingly being called upon to provide the highest-quality care, treatment, or services. This starts with effective, individualized treatment planning.

Tool 5-1. Plan for Care, Treatment, or Services Template

This sample template includes key points to consider when creating treatment plans. The Joint Commission does not require use of this template. It may be adapted and is offered as a way to capture information that should be included in your treatment plans based on your organization's policies as well as what is required by laws and federal regulations.

Tool 5-1. Plan for Care, Treatment, or Services Template	
Organization:	
Programs or Services:	
Date:	
DEMOGRAPHICS	
Individual Name:	Prefers to Be Called:
Primary or Preferred Language: ☐ English ☐Spanish ☐ Other:	
Preferred Method of Communication: ☐ Oral ☐ Written ☐ Sign Language	
Date of Birth:	Country of Birth:
Birth Gender: ☐ Male ☐ Female Gender Identification: Preferred pronouns:	Race/Ethnicity:
Address:	City:
State:	Zip:
Phone:	E-mail:
Marital/Relationship Status: ☐ Single (never married)____ ☐ Married–Years:____ ☐ Partnered–Years:____ ☐ Dating–Years:____ ☐ Divorced–Years Married:____ ☐ Separated–Years Married:____ ☐ Widowed–Years Married:____	
Family/Guardian: ☐ N/A	Family/Guardian Contact (phone/e-mail): ☐ N/A
Emergency Contact: ☐ N/A	Emergency Contact (phone/e-mail): ☐ N/A
CLINICAL/CASE MANAGEMENT	
Clinical/Case Record: ☐ Not Yet Created	Last Plan Update–Date: ☐ N/A
Authorized Staff:	
Admission or Entry–Date:	
Reason for Care, Treatment, or Services:	
Referral Source: ☐ N/A	Referral Contact (phone/e-mail): ☐ N/A

PRESENTING ISSUES
What happened to cause admission or entry?
Why admit or enter now?
Who referred the individual?

SOURCES OF INFORMATION	
Individuals	
☐ Individual ☐ Family/Guardian ☐ Significant Other(s) ☐ Licensed Mental Health Counselor (LMHC) ☐ Licensed Practitioner of the Healing Arts (LPHA) ☐ Licensed Mental Health Professional (LMHP) ☐ Psychiatrist ☐ Physician ☐ Social Worker ☐ Qualified Mental Health Professional (QMHP) ☐ Case Manager ☐ Other Providers:	
Documentation	
☐ Clinical/Case Record—Date: ☐ Risk of Harm Screening Form—Date: ☐ Suicide Risk Assessment Form—Date: ☐ N/A ☐ Medication Reconciliation Form—Date: ☐ Strength Assessment Questionnaire—Date: ☐ Spiritual Assessment Questionnaire—Date: ☐ Behavioral/Emotional Assessment Form—Date: ☐ Physical Pain Assessment Questionnaire—Date: ☐ Physical Health Screening Form—Date: ☐ Physical Health Examination Form—Date: ☐ N/A	☐ Diagnostic Summary Form—Date: ☐ Statement of Needs Form—Date: ☐ Coping Strategies Preferences Form—Date: ☐ Plan of Care, Treatment, or Services—Dates: ☐ Progress Note Form—Dates: ☐ Plan Review Form—Dates: ☐ Discharge Summary—Date: ☐ N/A ☐ Recovery Safety Plan—Date:

NEEDS, STRENGTHS, PREFERENCES, AND GOALS	
Needs *(caused by issues that may or may not be clinical)*	
Need 1:	☐ Active/Defined—Date: ☐ Deferred—Date: ☐ Referred—Date:
Need 2:	☐ Active/Defined—Date: ☐ Deferred—Date: ☐ Referred—Date:
Need 3:	☐ Active/Defined—Date: ☐ Deferred—Date: ☐ Referred—Date:
Strengths *(skills, talents, positive characteristics, and support to achieve goals for care, treatment, or services)*	
Preferences *(medication, counseling, and involvement of family/friends in care, treatment, or services)*	

Page **2** of **9**

Goals *(long-term; based on needs)*	
Need 1 *(from above)*:	
Goal 1:	☐ Defined—Date: ☐ Projected—Date: ☐ Achieved—Date:
Objective 1.1:	☐ Defined—Date: ☐ Projected—Date: ☐ Achieved—Date:

Interventions

☐ Assertiveness Training	☐ Pattern Identification and Interruption
☐ Anger Management	☐ Problem-Solving Skills Training
☐ Affect Identification and Expression	☐ Self/Other Boundaries Training
☐ Cognitive Restructuring	☐ Solution-Focused Techniques
☐ Communication Training	☐ Stress Management
☐ Decision Option Exploration	☐ Supportive Therapy
☐ Grief Work	☐ Family Therapy
☐ Imagery/Relaxation Training	☐ Group Therapy
☐ Medication Management	☐ Individual Therapy
☐ Meetings (see below)	☐ Other:
☐ Parent Training	

Meetings

☐ Alcoholics Anonymous (AA) ☐ Al-Anon ☐ Emotions Anonymous (EA) ☐ Narcotics Anonymous (NA)
☐ Overeaters Anonymous (OA) / Anorexics and Bulimics Anonymous (ABA)
☐ Self-Injury Recovery Anonymous (SIRA) ☐ Sex and Love Addicts Anonymous (SLAA)

☐ Obtain Sponsor ☐ Contact Sponsor—Times per Week:____ ☐ Attend Multifamily Group

Frequency: ☐ Daily ☐ Every Other Day ☐ 1–3 Times Weekly ☐ N/A ☐ Other:

Duration: ☐ 1 Week ☐ 2–4 Weeks ☐ Throughout Treatment ☐ N/A ☐ Other:

Staff Responsible:

Reviewed—Date: Reason for Review: Explanation of Any Changes:	Reviewed—Date: Reason for Review: Explanation of Any Changes:
Objective 1.2:	☐ Defined—Date: ☐ Projected—Date: ☐ Achieved—Date:

Interventions

☐ Assertiveness Training ☐ Anger Management ☐ Affect Identification and Expression ☐ Cognitive Restructuring ☐ Communication Training ☐ Decision Option Exploration ☐ Grief Work ☐ Imagery/Relaxation Training ☐ Medication Management ☐ Meetings (see below) ☐ Parent Training	☐ Pattern Identification and Interruption ☐ Problem-Solving Skills Training ☐ Self/Other Boundaries Training ☐ Solution-Focused Techniques ☐ Stress Management ☐ Supportive Therapy ☐ Family Therapy ☐ Group Therapy ☐ Individual Therapy ☐ Other:
Meetings ☐ AA ☐ Al-Anon ☐ EA ☐ NA ☐ OA / ABA ☐ SIRA ☐ SLAA ☐ Obtain Sponsor ☐ Contact Sponsor—Times per Week:____ ☐ Attend Multifamily Group	
Frequency: ☐ Daily ☐ Every Other Day ☐ 1–3 Times Weekly ☐ N/A ☐ Other: Duration: ☐ 1 Week ☐ 2–4 Weeks ☐ Throughout Treatment ☐ N/A ☐ Other:	
Staff Responsible:	
Reviewed—Date: Reason for Review: Explanation of Any Changes:	Reviewed—Date: Reason for Review: Explanation of Any Changes:
Need 2 *(from above)*:	
Goal 2	☐ Defined—Date: ☐ Projected—Date: ☐ Achieved—Date:
Objective 2.1:	☐ Defined—Date: ☐ Projected—Date: ☐ Achieved—Date:

Interventions

☐ Assertiveness Training	☐ Pattern Identification and Interruption
☐ Anger Management	☐ Problem-Solving Skills Training
☐ Affect Identification and Expression	☐ Self/Other Boundaries Training
☐ Cognitive Restructuring	☐ Solution-Focused Techniques
☐ Communication Training	☐ Stress Management
☐ Decision Option Exploration	☐ Supportive Therapy
☐ Grief Work	☐ Family Therapy
☐ Imagery/Relaxation Training	☐ Group Therapy
☐ Medication Management	☐ Individual Therapy
☐ Meetings (see below)	☐ Other:
☐ Parent Training	

Meetings

☐ AA ☐ Al-Anon ☐ EA ☐ NA ☐ OA / ABA ☐ SIRA ☐ SLAA

☐ ☐ Obtain Sponsor ☐ Contact Sponsor—Times per Week:____ ☐ Attend Multifamily Group

Frequency: ☐ Daily ☐ Every Other Day ☐ 1–3 Times Weekly ☐ N/A ☐ Other:

Duration: ☐ 1 Week ☐ 2–4 Weeks ☐ Throughout Treatment ☐ N/A ☐ Other:

Staff Responsible:

Reviewed—Date: Reason for Review: Explanation of Any Changes:	Reviewed—Date: Reason for Review: Explanation of Any Changes:
Objective 2.2:	☐ Defined—Date: ☐ Projected—Date: ☐ Achieved—Date:

Interventions

☐ Assertiveness Training	☐ Pattern Identification and Interruption
☐ Anger Management	☐ Problem-Solving Skills Training
☐ Affect Identification and Expression	☐ Self/Other Boundaries Training
☐ Cognitive Restructuring	☐ Solution-Focused Techniques
☐ Communication Training	☐ Stress Management
☐ Decision Option Exploration	☐ Supportive Therapy
☐ Grief Work	☐ Family Therapy
☐ Imagery/Relaxation Training	☐ Group Therapy
☐ Medication Management	☐ Individual Therapy
☐ Meetings (see below)	☐ Other:
☐ Parent Training	

Meetings

☐ AA ☐ Al-Anon ☐ EA ☐ NA ☐ OA / ABA ☐ SIRA ☐ SLAA

☐ ☐ Obtain Sponsor ☐ Contact Sponsor—Times per Week:____ ☐ Attend Multifamily Group

Frequency: ☐ Daily ☐ Every Other Day ☐ 1–3 Times Weekly ☐ N/A ☐ Other:

Duration: ☐ 1 Week ☐ 2–4 Weeks ☐ Throughout Treatment ☐ N/A ☐ Other:

Staff Responsible:

Reviewed—Date: Reason for Review: Explanation of Any Changes:	Reviewed—Date: Reason for Review: Explanation of Any Changes:
Objective 2.3:	☐ Defined—Date: ☐ Projected—Date: ☐ Achieved—Date:

Interventions

☐ Assertiveness Training
☐ Anger Management
☐ Affect Identification and Expression
☐ Cognitive Restructuring
☐ Communication Training
☐ Decision Option Exploration
☐ Grief Work
☐ Imagery/Relaxation Training
☐ Medication Management
☐ Meetings (see below)
☐ Parent Training
☐ Pattern Identification and Interruption
☐ Problem-Solving Skills Training
☐ Self/Other Boundaries Training
☐ Solution-Focused Techniques
☐ Stress Management
☐ Supportive Therapy
  ☐ Family Therapy
  ☐ Group Therapy
  ☐ Individual Therapy
☐ Other:

Meetings

☐ AA ☐ Al-Anon ☐ EA ☐ NA ☐ OA / ABA ☐ SIRA ☐ SLAA

☐ ☐ Obtain Sponsor ☐ Contact Sponsor—Times per Week:____ ☐ Attend Multifamily Group

Frequency: ☐ Daily ☐ Every Other Day ☐ 1–3 Times Weekly ☐ N/A ☐ Other:

Duration: ☐ 1 Week ☐ 2–4 Weeks ☐ Throughout Treatment ☐ N/A ☐ Other:

Staff Responsible:

Reviewed—Date: Reason for Review: Explanation of Any Changes:	Reviewed—Date: Reason for Review: Explanation of Any Changes:
Need 3 *(from above)*:	
Goal 3	☐ Defined—Date: ☐ Projected—Date: ☐ Achieved—Date:
Objective 3.1	☐ Defined—Date: ☐ Projected—Date: ☐ Achieved—Date:

Interventions

☐ Assertiveness Training
☐ Anger Management
☐ Affect Identification and Expression
☐ Cognitive Restructuring
☐ Communication Training
☐ Decision Option Exploration
☐ Grief Work
☐ Imagery/Relaxation Training
☐ Medication Management
☐ Meetings (see below)
☐ Parent Training
	☐ Pattern Identification and Interruption
	☐ Problem-Solving Skills Training
	☐ Self/Other Boundaries Training
	☐ Solution-Focused Techniques
	☐ Stress Management
	☐ Supportive Therapy
	  ☐ Family Therapy
	  ☐ Group Therapy
	  ☐ Individual Therapy
	☐ Other:

Meetings ☐ AA ☐ Al-Anon ☐ EA ☐ NA ☐ OA / ABA ☐ SIRA ☐ SLAA ☐ ☐ Obtain Sponsor ☐ Contact Sponsor—Times per Week:____ ☐ Attend Multifamily Group	
Frequency: ☐ Daily ☐ Every Other Day ☐ 1–3 Times Weekly ☐ N/A ☐ Other: Duration: ☐ 1 Week ☐ 2–4 Weeks ☐ Throughout Treatment ☐ N/A ☐ Other:	
Staff Responsible:	
Reviewed—Date: Reason for Review: Explanation of Any Changes:	Reviewed—Date: Reason for Review: Explanation of Any Changes:
MEDICATIONS	
Taking medications as ordered by prescriber? ☐ Yes ☐ No ☐ N/A (no prescriber-ordered medications)	
Prescription Medications	
Name: New: ☐ Yes ☐ No Dose: Frequency: Route: First Dose—Date: Last Dose—Date: Reason for Medication: Helpful? ☐ Yes ☐ No	Name: New: ☐ Yes ☐ No Dose: Frequency: Route: First Dose—Date: Last Dose—Date: Reason for Medication: Helpful? ☐ Yes ☐ No
Over-the-Counter Medications	
Name: New: ☐ Yes ☐ No Dose: Frequency: Route: First Dose—Date:	Name: New: ☐ Yes ☐ No Dose: Frequency: Route: First Dose—Date:

Last Dose—Date: Reason for Medication: Helpful? ☐ Yes ☐ No	Last Dose—Date: Reason for Medication: Helpful? ☐ Yes ☐ No
Vitamins, Supplements, Herbals, and Other	
Name: New: ☐ Yes ☐ No Dose: Frequency: Route: First Dose—Date: Last Dose—Date: Reason for Medication: Helpful? ☐ Yes ☐ No	Name: New: ☐ Yes ☐ No Dose: Frequency: Route: First Dose—Date: Last Dose—Date: Reason for Medication: Helpful? ☐ Yes ☐ No
Compliance and Education	
Taking medications as ordered by prescriber? ☐ Yes ☐ No ☐ N/A (no prescriber-ordered medications)	
Knowledgeable about current medications? ☐ Yes ☐ No	
Provided education on medications, as needed? ☐ Yes ☐ No	
Pharmacy	
Pharmacy:	Website:
Address:	City:
Phone:	☐ 24-hour ☐ Hours:
HEALTH CARE EDUCATION PROVIDED	
☐ Access to Health Care ☐ Exercise ☐ Hydration ☐ Nutrition ☐ Medications	☐ Coughing/Sneezing Etiquette ☐ Hand Hygiene ☐ Personal Hygiene
DISCHARGE CRITERIA	
Criteria 1:	☐ Defined—Date: ☐ Projected—Date: ☐ Achieved—Date:
Reviewed—Date: Reason for Review: Explanation of Any Changes:	Reviewed—Date: Reason for Review: Explanation of Any Changes:
Criteria 2:	☐ Defined—Date: ☐ Projected—Date: ☐ Achieved—Date:

Reviewed—Date: Reason for Review: Explanation of Any Changes:	Reviewed—Date: Reason for Review: Explanation of Any Changes:
Recommendations for Continuity of Care, Treatment, or Services:	☐ Defined—Date: ☐ Projected—Date: ☐ Achieved—Date:
Reviewed—Date: Reason for Review: Explanation of Any Changes:	Reviewed—Date: Reason for Review: Explanation of Any Changes:

DIAGNOSIS/CONDITION and DISPOSITION	
Diagnosis	
Code:	☐ Mild ☐ Moderate ☐ Severe ☐ Individual Denies ☐ N/A
Code:	☐ Mild ☐ Moderate ☐ Severe ☐ Individual Denies ☐ N/A
Reviewed—Date: Reason for Review: Explanation of Any Changes:	Reviewed—Date: Reason for Review: Explanation of Any Changes:
Condition and Disposition	
Reviewed—Date: Reason for Review: Explanation of Any Changes:	Reviewed—Date: Reason for Review: Explanation of Any Changes:

ATTESTATION	
Individual Signature:	Date:
Family/Guardian/Significant Other(s) Signature: ☐ N/A	Date:
Counselor Signature:	Date:
QMHP/Supervisor Signature:	Date:
LPHA/Physician Signature:	Date:

Tool 5-2. Plan for Care Evaluation Checklist

DOWNLOAD

This checklist includes criteria for plans for care, treatment, or services. You can use it to evaluate the quality of your organization's plans. Answers to all questions should ideally be Y *for* Yes *(unless they aren't applicable). Note: The following criteria apply to all behavioral health care and human services (BHC) programs/settings, but some programs/settings may have other, more specific criteria.*

Organization: ______________________ Program/Setting: ______________________

Date of Review: __________ Reviewer: ______________________

Needs, Strengths, Preferences, Goals	**Y**	**N**	**N/A**	**Comments**
Does the plan describe and reflect the behaviors of the individual served that support the need for care, treatment, or services?				
Does the plan identify current needs, strengths, preferences, and goals of the individual served that will be addressed during care, treatment, or services?				
Does the plan identify current needs, strengths, preferences, and goals of the individual served that will be referred?				
Does the plan identify current needs, strengths, preferences, and goals of the individual served that will be deferred?				
Does the plan state why the care, treatment, or services are necessary?				
Does the plan state why the setting is appropriate?				
If appropriate, does the plan state why alternative care, treatment, or services are *not* considered appropriate?				
Goals, Objectives, and Interventions	**Y**	**N**	**N/A**	**Comments**
Are the goals based on specific needs, strengths, and preferences, as well as goals of the individual?				
Are the plan's goals and objectives realistic?				
Do the objectives identify steps to achieve goals?				
Do the objectives offer a means of assessing progress or achievement?				
Does the plan provide indexes of progress?				
Does the plan state the type of interventions?				
Does the plan state the frequency of interventions?				
Does the plan include only activities designed to occur in a time frame that meets the assessed needs of the individual served?				
Does the plan identify the sources of information used to develop it?				

Page **1** of **2**

Adaptability and Change	Y	N	N/A	Comments
Does the plan include anticipated changes for the individual served?				
Does the plan include an anticipated time frame for the achievement of objectives and goals?				
Can the plan be adapted according the changing needs, strengths, preferences, and goals of the individual served?				
Does the plan document reasons a goal or an objective is deferred (as applicable)?				
Does the plan identify what changes in the individual served would prompt a discharge or transfer (if applicable)?				
Does the plan state the condition of the individual served upon completion of the care, treatment, or services (if applicable)?				
Does the plan address the ongoing needs of the individual served (at transfer, at discharge, or for continuing care)?				
Does the plan identify factors that support the transition to community integration, when that is identified as a need?				
Language and Use	**Y**	**N**	**N/A**	**Comments**
Does the plan incorporate the words of the individual served as much as possible?				
Does the plan address involvement of the family/guardian and/or significant others (as appropriate)?				
Is the plan written in clear, plain language?				
Does the plan facilitate a team approach to providing care, treatment, or services (if applicable to the program/setting)?				

Page **2** of **2**

Glossary

addiction services Care, treatment, and services provided to individuals with substance use disorders or addictive behaviors.

aggregate data Measurement data collected and reported by organizations as a sum or total over a given time period (for example, monthly, quarterly) or for certain groupings (for example, health care organization level).

assessment The process established by the organization for obtaining clinically relevant information about each individual seeking human services or behavioral health care, treatment, or services. The information is used to match an individual's need with the appropriate setting, service/program, and intervention.

case management, or coordination Assistance provided to individuals or their authorized representatives aimed at assessing needs, linking community resources, coordinating services, and delivering flexible problem solving and crisis response.

case plan An individualized plan for or provision of services that addresses the needs, safety, and well-being of an individual while in foster care.

child welfare agency An organization that provides services designed to keep children safe and provide families with the support necessary to care for their children successfully.

data management The practice of managing data as a resource for identifying potential that involves strategies and reliable methods to access, integrate, store, and prepare data for analysis.

diagnostic summary, or summary statement A statement included in the comprehensive treatment plan that reflects and documents the clinician's analysis of screening and assessment data and identifies and prioritizes expressed needs to further develop the plan.

Generalized Anxiety Disorder-7 (GAD-7) Questionnaire A seven-question instrument designed to assess and monitor severity of generalized anxiety in an individual. When properly used, it complies with Joint Commission requirements. Each response to items in the GAD-7 is scored 0–3, with a total score range of 0–21. Specific ranges of scores reflect varying levels of anxiety severity (for example, scores of 0–5 indicate mild anxiety; scores of 15–21 indicate severe anxiety).

goals The achievable outcomes for treatment that are expressed by the individual served and identified in clear language; are built on the strengths of the individual served; and include measurable, time-bound objectives.

intensive outpatient program (IOP) Short-term, acute treatment program used to address addictions, depression, eating disorders, or other dependencies that do not require detoxification or round-the-clock supervision of the individual served. IOPs (also known as intensive outpatient treatment [IOT] programs) enable patients to continue with their normal, day-to-day lives (for example, live at home and continue to work) in a way that residential treatment programs do not.

interdisciplinary An approach to care, treatment, or services that involves two or more disciplines or professions (for example, social work, nursing, counselors who provided prior treatment, substance abuse counselors, spiritual support, psychology, psychiatry, legal advocate, case manager, probation officer, primary care providers, music, or art therapy) collaborating to plan, treat, or provide care, treatment, or services to an individual served and/or that person's family.

interventions Clinical tools used by the treatment team to help individuals achieve their goals and objectives.

measurement-based care Care, treatment, or services that use data gathered through screening and assessment to monitor the progress of the individual served, inform the individual's goals and objectives, and drive decisions about care. When successfully implemented, measurement-based care (sometimes referred to as *feedback-informed treatment* or *outcome-informed care*) benefits both the individual served and the organization that provides care, treatment or services to the individual.

motivational interviewing An evidence-based clinical technique designed to encourage individuals to talk themselves into making beneficial changes by using open-ended questions, affirming dialogue, reflective listening, and summarizing with an aim to cultivate individuals' belief in their own ability to grow and change.

multidimensional assessment An evidence-based approach to assessment for addiction that takes into account the needs, obstacles, and liabilities of individuals served, as well as their assets, resources, and personal support structure. Together, these are used to determine the appropriate level of care.

needs The basic necessities required to produce a good treatment outcome. The needs of individuals served should focus on the presenting problems identified by individuals that are relevant to their care.

objectives Actionable behaviors that help individuals reach their goals.

Patient Health Questionnaire-9 (PHQ-9) A nine-question instrument designed to assess and monitor levels of depression in an individual. When properly used, it complies with Joint Commission requirements. Each response to items in the PHQ-9 is scored 0–3, with a total score range of 0–27. Specific ranges of scores reflect varying levels of depression severity (for example, scores of 5–9 indicate mild depression; scores of 20–27 indicate severe depression).

permanency planning The US Department of Health and Human Services Child Welfare Information Gateway defines *permanency planning* as a systematic effort to provide long-term continuity in a dependent child's care, as an alternative to temporary foster placements. This might be done by facilitating adoption, by establishing clear guidelines for remaining in foster care, or by helping the child's family become capable of meeting the child's needs.

plan of care, treatment, or services See treatment plan.

preferences Factors that account for whether an individual will be actively engaged in treatment, such as the following: preference for appointment times and communication formats, language proficiency, cultural preferences, and so on.

reassessment Ongoing data collection that begins on initial assessment, comparing the most recent data collected with the data collected at the previous assessment.

resource family/parent A family/parent, other than the individual's family or parent of origin, who cares for the individual in the capacity of a primary parent. This could be a relative (kinship care), foster parent, respite caregiver, or adoptive parent.

scope of service The activities defined by the organization and permitted by relevant licensing authorities as descriptive of the services the organization provides.

screening Process of determining whether individuals have certain risk factors associated with physical or behavioral health issues requiring further assessment.

shared decision making In mental health, shared decision making is a process in which clinicians and patients work together to select tests, treatments, management, or support packages, based on clinical evidence and the individual's informed preferences. It involves the provision of evidence-based information about options, outcomes, and uncertainties, together with decision support counseling and a system for recording and implementing individuals' informed preferences.

strengths Factors that support the health and well-being of an individual and empower with positive purpose, including, for example, religious beliefs, support network of family/friends, ability to work or care for others, and capacity to hope.

trauma The Joint Commission defines *trauma* as an experience that creates a sense of fear, helplessness, or horror that overwhelms an individual's resources for coping.

trauma-Informed care An approach to care, treatment, and services that takes into account the impact of traumatic stress on an individual's sense of safety, ability to self-regulate, sense of self, perception of control and self-efficacy, and interpersonal relationships. Common experiences of trauma may include sexual abuse, physical abuse, severe neglect, loss, acts of violence, and/or the witnessing of violence, terrorism, and/or disasters.

treatment plan A written plan, based on data gathered during screening and assessment, that identifies care, treatment, or service needs, strengths, preferences, and goals; describes the strategy for meeting those needs, preferences, and goals; builds on the strengths and considers the preferences of the individual served; and documents progress toward meeting the plan's objectives. The plan may include care, treatment, habilitation, and rehabilitation.

Index

A

Abuse, neglect, and exploitation. *See also* Trauma
as examples of traumatic experiences, 21
screening for, 13
screening for and identification of individuals who may have experienced, 9–10, 13
Addiction services
appropriate level of care for individuals with, 64
assessment/multidimensional assessment for, 68
assessment of individual's addictive behaviors, 63–64
COVID-19 pandemic and increase in need for, 67
drug testing, staff education and training on, 64, 69
drug testing policy, 64, 69
goals for treatment, 69
individualized treatment plan development, 68–70
interventions and services to meet goals, 69
IOPs for provision of, 67
medical histories, physical exams, and diagnostic and laboratory testing, process for, 63
overdose and fatal overdose data, 67
requirements for, 66–67
screening and assessment for, 13, 37
screening and treatment planning for, 67–68
standards related to, 37, 63–64
testing and monitoring related to, 69
treatment outcomes and individual's readiness to change, 67–68
American Society of Addiction Medicine, ASAM Criteria/ASAM Patient Placement Criteria, 68
Ask Suicide-Screening Questions (ASQ) Brief Suicide Safety Assessment, 19
Ask Suicide-Screening Questions (ASQ) toolkit, 16–17, 19
Assessment and reassessment
addiction assessment/multidimensional assessment, 68
addictive behaviors, assessment of, 63–64
child welfare services, assessment for, 13, 14, 64, 70–71, 75–81
co-occurring disorders and scope of, 36
definition and purpose of, 12–13, 36–37
diagnostic summary/summary statement of data from, 37–38
evaluation of assessment strategies, 39–40
importance of, 5, 6–7
involvement of individual in, 38
nutritional screening triggers for additional assessment, 20
population-specific assessment, 13, 37
prioritizing needs for, 37–38

reassessment
importance and purpose of, 38–39
importance of, 36
monitoring outcomes and progress through, 38, 39, 54–55
requirements for, 35, 37
screening compared to assessment, 12–13
setting-specific assessment, 13, 36
successful strategies for, 39, 40
suicide assessment
evidence-based process for, 10, 16
monitoring implementation and effectiveness of policies and procedures for screening, assessment, and management of individuals at risk for suicide, 10, 16
tools for, 37, 39
treatment plan to address needs and problems identified in, 6, 35, 64

B

Behavioral Health Care and Human Services (BHC) program
compliance challenges identified during surveys of, 5–6, 11, 15–16, 20–21, 41–42, 44, 55–56
new and revised requirements for, 7, 66, 67, 70
types of organizations accredited under, 6, 37, 66–67, 73
Behavioral Healthcare Instruments Listing website, 55
Behavioral Health Home option, 6
Behavioral health issues, prevalence of, 5

C

Care, Treatment, and Services (CTS) standards
addictions, appropriate level of care for individuals with (CTS.02.03.13), 64
addictions treatment (CTS.02.03.07; CTS.02.03.13), 37, 63–64
assessment of individuals (CTS.03.01.03), 5–6, 23
assessment of individual's addictive behaviors (CTS.02.03.07), 63–64
assessment of individuals for child welfare services (CTS.02.04.01), 64, 70
children and youth, assessment of (CTS.02.03.03), 37
child welfare case plan, development and review of (CTS.03.02.03), 64–66, 70
chronic physical health conditions, management of (CTS.02.02.01), 37
compliance and noncompliance with requirements, 5–6, 20–21, 41–42, 44, 55–56, 90
drug testing policy (CTS.02.03.15), 64, 69
eating disorders treatment (CTS.02.03.09; CTS.02.03.11), 37
family involvement in plan for care, treatment, or services (CTS.03.01.05), 36, 46
intellectual and development disorders, assessment of individuals with (CTS.02.03.05), 37
measurement-based care (CTS.03.01.09), 38
medical histories, physical exams, and diagnostic and laboratory testing (CTS.02.02.09), 63
nutritional status, screening for (CTS.02.01.11), 9, 13, 20
opioid treatment programs (CTS.02.02.07; CTS.02.02.09), 37
outcomes of care, treatment, and services, monitoring and assessment of (CTS.03.01.09), 51, 52, 53, 55–56
physical pain, screening for (CTS.02.01.09), 9, 13
plan for care, treatment, or services reflects assessed needs of individual served (CTS.03.01.03), 5–6, 35, 64
planned care, treatment, or services based on needs, strengths, preferences, and goals of individual (CTS.03.01.01), 10
preliminary plan for care, treatment, or services, development of (CTS.01.03.01), 9, 12

referrals for additional care, treatment, or services not offered by organization (CTS.03.01.07), 36, 47
requirements for, 5
safety plan (CTS.01.03.01), 9
screening of individuals for child welfare services (CTS.02.04.01), 64, 70
screening procedure for early detection of risk of imminent harm to self or others (CTS.02.01.01), 9, 13
trauma, abuse, neglect, or exploitation, screening for and identification of individuals who may have experienced (CTS.02.02.05), 9–10, 13
Care, treatment, or services. *See also* Plan of care, treatment, or services/treatment plan
frequency of interventions and services, 7, 11
interventions and services to meet goals, 7, 11, 14, 43, 45–46
provision according to treatment plan, 35
provision of and meeting needs of individuals, 5
scope of services and treatment plan development, 11
Case samples and treatment plans
depression and grief/loss example, 83–87
substance abuse example, 88–89
Center for Health Care Strategies trauma-informed care strategies, 21–23
Center for Substance Abuse Treatment (CSAT) Treatment Improvement Protocols (TIPs), 70
Centers for Disease Control and Prevention, US (CDC), 67
Child and Adolescent Needs and Strengths (CANS) too, 71, 75–81
Children and youth, assessment of, 37
Child welfare/child welfare agencies
after-care planning, 73
case plan, definition and information included in, 70
case planning requirements for, 67
case plans for, development and review of, 7, 64–66, 70
cultural and age-specific competence of staff, 66, 71
new and revised requirements for, 66, 70
performance improvement priorities, 52
permanency goal and planning, 65, 71–72
plan for care, treatment, or services reflects assessed needs of individual served, 64
reunification or permanency options assessment, 65, 72
review and revision of case plan, 73
screening and assessment for, 13, 14, 64, 70–71, 75–81
staff education, training, and competence for job responsibilities, 66, 71
standards related to, 64–66, 70
tools for screening and assessment, 71, 75–81
transitional living and independence preparations and planning, 65, 72, 73
trauma-informed assessment, 64, 70–71
trauma-informed case plan, 70–71
trauma screening, 22–23
Collaborative and interdisciplinary care, treatment, or services
needs, strengths, preferences, and goals of individual as basis for treatment plan, 10, 42–43, 45
process for, 7, 11
Columbia-Suicide Severity Rating Scale (C-SSRS) Triage version tool, 17, 19
Community, support for recovery from, 5, 69
Comprehensive Accreditation Manual for Behavioral Health Care and Human Services (*CAMBHC*)
special population and program requirements in, 6, 37, 66–67, 73
Standards Applicability Process (SAP) chapter, 6, 66–67
updates to standards and requirements in, 7, 66, 67, 70

Core Set of Outcome Measures for Behavioral Health Across Service Settings, A (Kennedy Forum), 55
Counseling and follow-up care
  written policies and procedures to address care of individuals at risk for suicide, 10
COVID-19 pandemic
  addiction and substance use disorders related to, 67
  behavioral health care demand related to, 5, 90
  suicide ideation related to, prevalence of, 15
C-SSRS (Columbia-Suicide Severity Rating Scale) Triage version tool, 17, 19
Cultural and age-specific staff competence, 66, 71
Cultural beliefs, 14

D

Daily activities and daily living skills
  purpose and engagement in, 5
  screening process and identification of strengths related to, 14
Data collection and analysis
  aggregation and analysis of data to evaluate and monitor progress, 51, 55, 56
  compliance and noncompliance with requirements, 55–56
  outcome measurement tracer questions, 56, 62
  quality and performance improvement, data use for, 52, 56
  requirements for, 51, 52
  standards related to, 51, 52
Data management assessment and reviews, 56
Deferrals. *See* Referrals and deferrals
Deferred goals, 44–45
Depression
  assessment for, 36
  case sample and treatment plan, 83–87
  disability related to, 5
  divorce and example of treatment for, 14
  identification through screening process, 13
  IOPs for provision of treatment to address, 67
  Patient Health Questionnaire-9 (PHQ-9) Depression Scale
    aggregation and analysis of data from, 55
    case sample and treatment plan, 84–86
    description and scoring of, 18, 39, 54
    repeated administration and frequency of use of, 39, 53
    sample of, 48
    sharing results with individual, 54–55
Discharge or transfer, planning for, 6
Drug testing policy, 64, 69

E

Eating disorders
  data collection as basis for assessment of outcomes of care, treatment, and services, 51
  IOPs for provision of treatment to address, 67
  screening and assessment for, 13, 20, 36, 37
ED-SAFE Study Materials, 20
Environment/physical spaces

environmental risk assessment, 10, 16
ligature-resistant environments, 16
safe environment for individuals who have experienced trauma, 22
Ethical business practices (LD.04.02.03), 66
Exploitation. *See* Abuse, neglect, and exploitation

F

Faith or religious beliefs, 14
Families
involvement in treatment planning and plan, 36, 46
reunification or permanency options assessment, 65, 72
screening process and identification of strengths related to, 14
support for recovery from, 5
Feedback-informed treatment, 52. *See also* Measurement-based care
Friends
addiction services and IOP goals related to, 69
screening process and identification of strengths related to, 14

G

Generalized Anxiety Disorder-7 (GAD-7) Questionnaire, 39, 49
Glossary, 103–105
Goals for care, treatment, or services
addiction services and IOP treatment goals, 69
checklist to evaluate treatment plan for, 100–101
child welfare case plan inclusion of, 64–66
compliance and noncompliance with requirements, 5–6, 41–42, 44
deferred goals, 44–45
definition and individualized nature of, 14
examples of, 41
identification through assessment, 35, 41
individualized goals and objectives, 6, 35, 41
interventions and services to meet, 7, 11, 14, 43, 45–46, 69
measurable goals and objectives, 6, 7, 11, 14, 41, 42
monitoring outcomes and progress to achieve goals, 6, 7, 11, 38, 39, 41, 51, 54–56
multiple interventions for, 45–46
objectives to achieve goals, 41
permanency goal and planning, 65, 71–72
priority of goals, 44–45
progress toward meeting, 6
review and revision of, 6, 7, 11, 35, 43–44, 54
scripted language for, 6, 11, 42
successful strategies for, 41, 42
words and ideas of individual in statements of, 5, 7, 11, 14, 35, 41, 42

H

Health/physical health
assessment process and referrals for medical treatment, 37
chronic physical health conditions, management of, 37
medical histories, physical exams, and diagnostic and laboratory testing, process for, 63

medical history and physical exam, 15
physical pain, screening for, 9, 13, 15
recovery and healthy choices that support, 5
screening for physical health, 13, 15
Human Resources Management (HRM) standards
staff competence to perform job responsibilities and duties (HRM.01.06.01), 66, 71
staff education and training (HRM.01.05.01), 66, 71

I

Individualized treatment plan
addiction services and IOP treatment plans, 67–70
compliance and noncompliance with requirements, 6, 90
requirements for, 11, 90
scripted language for, 6, 11, 42
Intellectual and development disorders, individuals with
screening and assessment of, 13, 14, 37
Intensive outpatient programs (IOPs)
co-occurring issues and retention rate, 69
goals for treatment, 69
individualized treatment plan development, 68–70
interventions and services to meet goals, 69
length of stay in, 68–69
referrals to, 68
requirements for, 67
screening and treatment planning for, 67–68
service recommendations from SAMHSA for, 69
services provided by, 67
testing and monitoring during treatment in, 69
treatment outcomes and individual's readiness to change, 67–68
Interdisciplinary treatment plans. *See* Collaborative and interdisciplinary care, treatment, or services

K

Kennedy Forum, 55

L

Leadership (LP) standards
ethical business practices (LD.04.02.03), 66
performance improvement priorities (LD.03.07.01), 52
Ligature-resistant environments, 16

M

Malnutrition, 20, 37
Measurement-based care
benefits of, 52, 57
compliance and noncompliance with requirements, 55–56
data collection and analysis
aggregation and analysis of data to evaluate and monitor progress, 51, 55, 56
compliance and noncompliance with requirements, 55–56
requirements for, 51, 52
standards related to, 51, 52

data management assessment and reviews, 56
definition of, 52
measurable goals and objectives, 6, 7, 11, 14
monitoring outcomes and progress through reassessment, 38, 39, 54–55
outcome improvement through, 7, 52
outcome measurement tracer questions, 56, 62
outcome measures, core set of, 55
outcomes of care, treatment, and services measurement procedure policy template, 55, 58–61
outcomes of care, treatment, and services, monitoring and assessment of, 51, 52, 55–56
policies and procedures for, 52, 55
staff training on use and benefit of measurement tools, 55–56
standard related to, 38
tool or instrument to assess outcomes of care, 52, 53
criteria for selection of, 53
listing of and resources related to, 55
Medical history and physical exam, 15, 63
Mock tracer activities, 56, 62
Motivational interviewing, 42, 67, 68

N

National Action Alliance for Suicide Prevention, Recommended Standard Care for People with Suicide Risk report, 19
National Alliance on Mental Illness, data on mental health treatment from, 5
National Institute of Mental Health (NIMH)
Ask Suicide-Screening Questions (ASQ) toolkit, 16–17
ED-SAFE Study Materials, 20
National Patient Safety Goal (NPSG)
compliance and noncompliance with requirements, 15–16
suicide risk, reduction of (NPSG.15.01.01), 10, 13, 15
Needs, strengths, preferences, and goals of individual. *See also* Goals for care, treatment, or services
as basis for treatment plan, 10, 11, 35, 42–43, 45
checklist to evaluate treatment plan for, 100
child welfare screening and assessment to identify, 71, 75–81
goals, definition and individualized nature of, 14
identification through assessment, 35, 37–38, 64
identification through screening, 12–15
needs, definition and role in treatment outcome, 13
preferences
definition and influence in treatment, 14
planned interventions and consideration of, 45, 46
strengths, definition and development of objectives and interventions in plan, 13–14
Neglect. *See* Abuse, neglect, and exploitation
Nutritional status, screening for, 9, 13, 20

O

Opioid treatment programs, 6, 37
Outcome-informed treatment, 52. *See also* Measurement-based care
Outcome measurement tracer questions, 56, 62
Outcome measures, core set of, 55

P

Pain, screening for, 9, 13, 15
Patient Health Questionnaire-9 (PHQ-9) Depression Scale
  aggregation and analysis of data from, 55
  case sample and treatment plan, 84–86
  description and scoring of, 18, 39, 54
  repeated administration and frequency of use of, 39, 53
  sample of, 48
  sharing results with individual, 54–55
Pediatric suicide risk screening, clinical pathways to address, 19
Performance improvement
  data use for quality and performance improvement, 52, 56
  priorities for, 52
Performance Improvement (PI) standards
  data collection and analysis (PI.03.01.01), 52
Permanency goal and planning, 65, 71–72
Policies and procedures
  drug testing policy, 64, 69
  evaluation and improvement of, 55, 89–90
  measurement-based care policies and procedures, 52, 55
  outcomes of care, treatment, and services measurement procedure policy template, 55, 58–61
  plan of care development policy template, 11, 24–34
  review of screening practices, policies, and procedures, 15
  screening processes, 14–15
  suicide risk
    monitoring implementation and effectiveness of policies and procedures for screening, assessment, and management of individuals at risk for suicide, 10
    written policies and procedures to address care of individuals at risk for suicide, 10
Preferences. *See* Needs, strengths, preferences, and goals of individual

Q

Quality and performance improvement, data use for, 52, 56

R

Recommended Standard Care for People with Suicide Risk report, 19
Record of Care, Treatment, and Services (RC) standards
  audit of clinical/case records (RC.01.04.01), 90
Recovery
  definition of, 5
  support for life in, 5
Recovery Village, The, 67
Referrals and deferrals
  IOPs, referrals to, 68
  process for and documentation of, 36, 46–47
  requirements for, 7, 11, 47
Religious beliefs or faith, 14

S

Safety plan, 9
Satisfaction surveys, 55
SBQ-R (Suicide Behavior Questionnaire-Revised), 18
Screening individuals
addiction services and IOPs screening process, 67–68
assessment compared to screening, 12–13
child welfare services, screening for, 13, 14, 64, 70–71, 75–81
compliance and noncompliance with requirements, 20–21
effectiveness of processes for, 14–15
harm to self or others, screening procedures for detection of, 9, 13
importance of, 5, 6, 23
needs, strengths, preferences, and goals identification through screening, 12–15
nutritional status, screening for, 9, 13, 20
policies and procedures on and processes for, 12, 14–15
population-specific screening, 13
review of screening practices, policies, and procedures, 15
self-reported data as part of, 14–15
setting-specific screening, 13
staff competence for, 13, 15
standards related to, 9–10
suicide risk, screening for, 6, 13, 15–20
evidence-based process to identify level of risk, 13, 15
monitoring implementation and effectiveness of policies and procedures for screening, assessment, and management of individuals at risk for suicide, 10, 16
suicidal ideation, screening for, 10, 13, 15
validated screening tools to identify risk, 13, 15, 16–20
trauma, screening for, 6, 9–10, 13, 21, 22–23
treatment plan to address needs and problems identified in, 6
Shared decision making, 43
Staff
competence to perform screening processes, 13, 15
cultural and age-specific competence of, 66, 71
drug testing, education and training on, 64, 69
measurement tools, training on use and benefit of, 55–56
secondary traumatic stress among, prevention of, 22
standards related to education, training, and competence of, 66, 71
suicide risk screening, staff training and competence for, 15
trauma-specific care, training for, 21–22, 23, 71
Standards Applicability Process (SAP) chapter, 6, 66–67
Strengths. *See* Needs, strengths, preferences, and goals of individual
Substance Abuse and Mental Health Services Administration (SAMHSA)
Center for Substance Abuse Treatment (CSAT) Treatment Improvement Protocols (TIPs), 70
IOP data from, 68–69
IOP service recommendations from, 69
Substance use disorders. *See also* Addiction services
assessment for, 36
case sample and treatment plan, 88–89
COVID-19 pandemic and increase in need for, 67

goals for treatment, 69
interventions and services to meet goals, 69
IOPs for provision of treatment to address, 67
overdose and fatal overdose data, 67
requirements for treatment of, 7
screening and treatment planning for, 67–68
screening process and needs of individual, 13
testing and monitoring related to, 69
treatment planning for, 7
Suicide Behavior Questionnaire-Revised (SBQ-R), 18
Suicide risk
assessment of individuals, 10, 16
compliance and noncompliance with screening requirements for, 15–16
documentation of level of risk, 10
environmental risk assessment to minimize risks, 10, 16
evidence-based process to identify level of risk, 13, 15
mitigation of risk for suicide, 10, 15–16
monitoring implementation and effectiveness of policies and procedures for screening, assessment, and management of individuals at risk for suicide, 10, 16
National Patient Safety Goal on reduction of, 10, 13, 15
screening for, 6, 13, 15–20
staff training and competence related to screening for, 15
suicidal ideation, screening for, 10, 13, 15
validated screening tools to identify, 13, 15, 16–20
written policies and procedures to address care of individuals at risk for suicide, 10

T

Tools, 7
access to, 8
Child and Adolescent Needs and Strengths (CANS) tool, 71, 75–81
Generalized Anxiety Disorder-7 (GAD-7) Questionnaire, 39, 49
measurement-based tools and instruments, listing of and resources related to, 55
Patient Health Questionnaire-9 (PHQ-9) Depression Scale
aggregation and analysis of data from, 55
case sample and treatment plan, 84–86
description and scoring of, 18, 39, 54
repeated administration and frequency of use of, 39, 53
sample of, 48
sharing results with individual, 54–55
plan of care development policy template, 11, 24–34
suicide prevention screening tools, 13, 15, 16–20
treatment plan template, 89, 91–99
Tracer questions for mock tracer activities, 56, 62
Transitional living and independence preparations and planning, 65, 72, 73
Trauma
abuse, neglect, and exploitation as examples of, 21
assessment, trauma-informed, 64, 70–71
child welfare case plan, trauma-informed, 70–71
definition of, 21

effects of, 21
evidence-based trauma-specific treatment approaches, 23
rescreening and revisiting traumatic experience, 23
safe environment for individuals who have experienced, 22
screening for, 6, 9–10, 13, 21, 22–23
staff training for interacting with individuals who have experienced, 21–22, 23, 71
strategies for trauma-informed care, 21–23
tools for screening for, 22
Trauma-Focused Cognitive Behavioral Therapy (TF-CBT), 23
Treatment plan/plan of care, treatment, or services. *See also* Individualized treatment plan; Needs, strengths, preferences, and goals of individual
addiction services and IOP treatment plans, 67–70
assessment as basis for, 35, 64
collaborative and interdisciplinary treatment plans, 10, 42–43, 45
compliance and noncompliance with requirements, 5–6, 11, 44, 90
decision making for, individual involvement in, 6, 11, 22
definition of, 11
evaluation of plan
activities from, 89–90
checklist for, 90, 100–101
failure to follow written plan, 6
family involvement in, 36, 46
importance of, 5
preliminary plan of care, 9, 11, 12
provision of care, treatment, or services according to, 35
review and revision of, 43–44, 54
sample plan of care development policy, 11, 24–34
scope of services and development of, 11
standards related to, 9–10, 35–36
trauma-informed care, strategies for integration into, 21–23
unique treatment settings and services, 7, 66–67
written treatment plans
case samples and treatment plans, 83–88
development of and elements in, 89, 91–99

W

World Health Organization, data on depression from, 5